My Memories of World War II

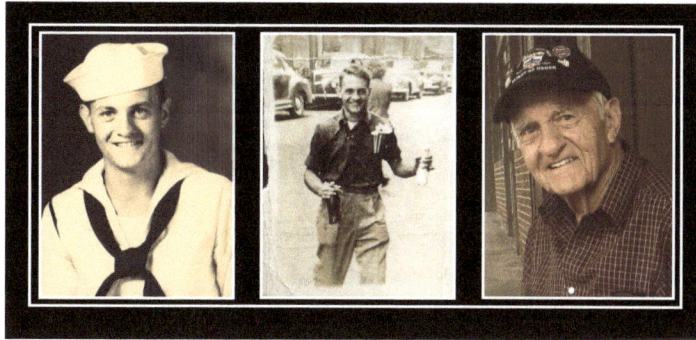

James E. Brooks
Author

Stephanie Fairchild Fister
Collaborator, Editor

Dedicated to the men and women who gave their lives
in the fight against tyranny during WWII...

and to young people in the hope they can learn the
lessons of WWII to prevent similar
global tragedies in the future.

What's Best for Our Kids
        Publishing

First printing: 2015
Printed with Dyslexie, a font designed to make
reading faster, easier, and more enjoyable for all readers,
especially those with dyslexia.
Library of Congress Cataloging-in-publication Data
Fister, Stephanie Fairchild
ISBN 978-0-9740064-1-3
James E.Brooks, Author
Stephanie Fairchild Fister, Editor

    1. WWII History
    2. Education
    3. Font for Dyslexia
Printed in the United States of America

The words in this book are the memories of
James E. Brooks who served in the Navy during World War II.

He shared his memories aloud with his niece Stephanie
as she wrote down what he wanted to convey about his experiences.

The first time I left my hometown of Harlan, Kentucky was the day I was drafted for World War II. It was 1942 and I had just turned 18 years old. The war had already been going on in Europe, Africa, and Asia for seven years. The United States had been in the war for only a year when I entered.

The draft, at the time, started for boys at the age of 18, so it was my time to go. I was still in high school. I said goodbye to my family, friends, and teachers, packed a few things and left Harlan on a bus with other boys my age.

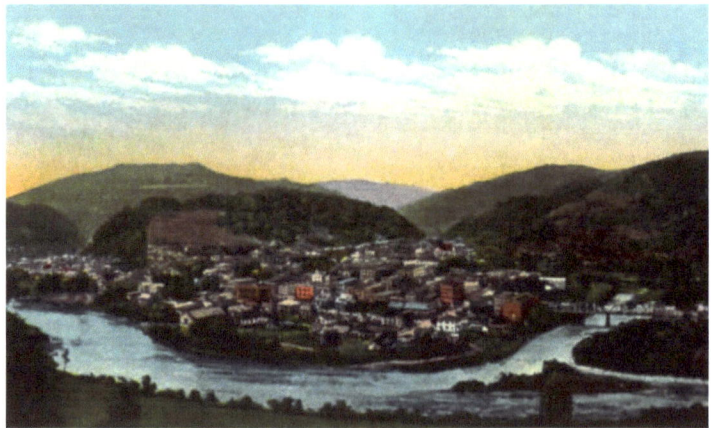
Harlan KY

Everyone in Harlan worried for the boys in our town as we each got older and the war drug on and on. When each young man turned 18 his mother and father would naturally feel sad and dreaded seeing their son go to war. There was an uneasiness for everyone because many of our soldiers were being killed overseas day after day and no one knew how the war might end.

After each son left for war, their return home was constantly on the minds of those who loved them. Families waited eagerly for letters and information concerning the safety of sons, nephews, and neighbors. There were women who went too. Women were not permitted to be soldiers then. They worked as nurses, technicians and other important jobs, all of us doing our best to defeat the enemy.

Each family worried, constantly hoping their loved one would survive until the war was over; never knowing when the end of the war would come. News about each battle could be found in the newspapers, on the radio, and at the movie theaters. Everyone always looked for the latest news. The war was part of daily conversation for most Americans.

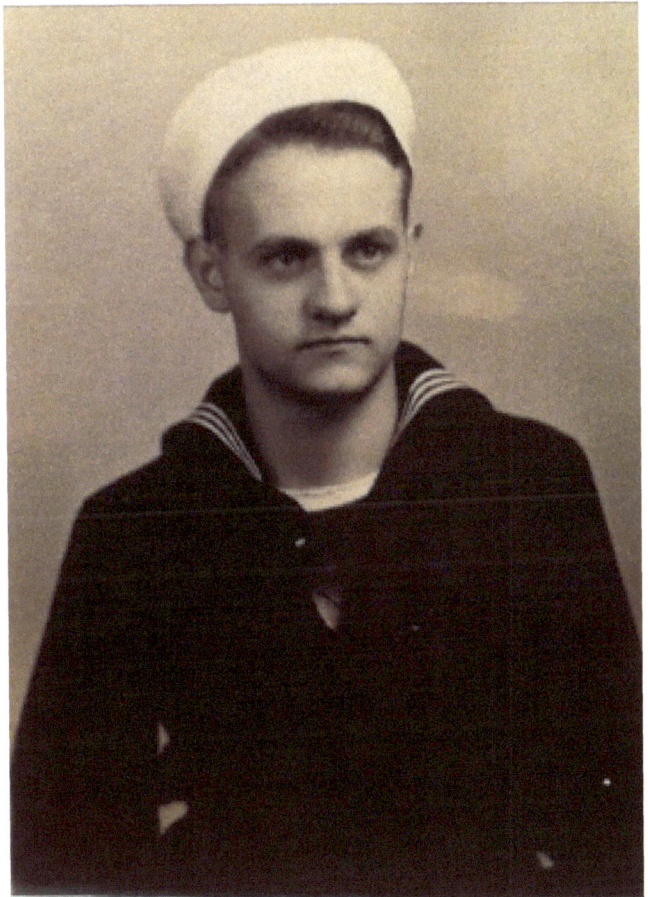

James E. Brooks

My father was a coal miner but he also was in charge of the post office for our small mountain community called Black Joe. He saw firsthand all the letters coming and going from soldiers and families. Our family also ran a boarding house where many coal miners lived. My mother cooked all their meals and even cleaned their rooms for them. I remember her packing their lunch pails before they left for the mines early each morning. Both my parents worked hard to give my sisters and me the food and clothes we needed. Things were not easy. We all worked hard.

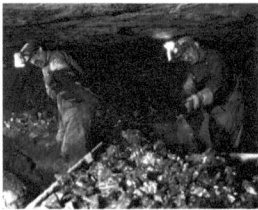

National Museum of American History

These photos are of coal miners in Eastern Kentucky. I remember my father and the men who boarded with us looking like this. They came home in the evening, worn out from chopping at coal in the dark mines all day. This picture must be at the beginning of the workday, I remember the whites of their eyes seemed so bright against their skin and clothes that had been covered in thick black coal dust. Most of them still had their oil-fuel lamp helmets on their heads when they got home.

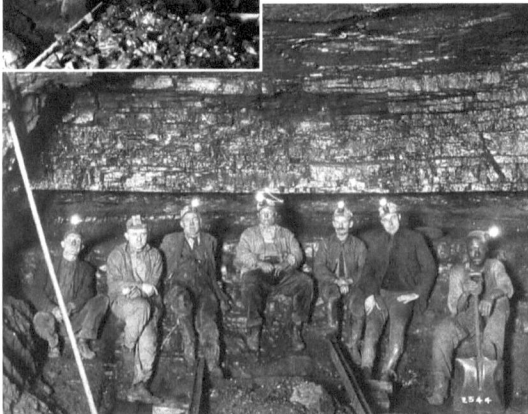

I remember once, when I was very young, I thought I would help the men who were boarding with us while they were out working in the mines. I went in each of their rooms and broke each of their cigarettes in half. I thought it would give them double the amount of cigarettes! I couldn't have been more than four years old. The miners, along with my father, were not happy with me for doing this. I learned quickly that the cigarettes I broke were ruined. After a long talk with Mother and Dad they understood that I did not mean to be bad and that I was actually trying to help. Now that we know cigarettes are bad for us I guess I was doing a good thing after all, but we didn't know that at the time. We've learned so much about lung health since then!

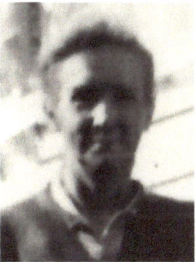

Despite the conflicts between the coal companies and the unions, most days were pleasant and we enjoyed being with our family and friends. We didn't know we were poor. There were songs and stories to listen to on the radio, and Mother's food was delicious. Her chicken and dumplings and fried chicken were especially good. Everyone loved and complimented her cooking. As I look back on her life, I wonder how she did all that she did for our family and the miners. We didn't know what was about to happen to our world.

My parents knew very little of world events and politics of our time. Life for us was about living day to day in our town. I believe this was true for most people in the 1930s and 40s. Families were still recovering from the Great Depression when many people lost their life's savings due to problems with the economy and the banking system. To make things worse, a crisis called the Dust Bowl had just devastated the western states. Fields that had been overly planted year after year became dry and the wind created massive storms of dust that ruined farms. Many families who lost their farms had to move to find work in order to survive.

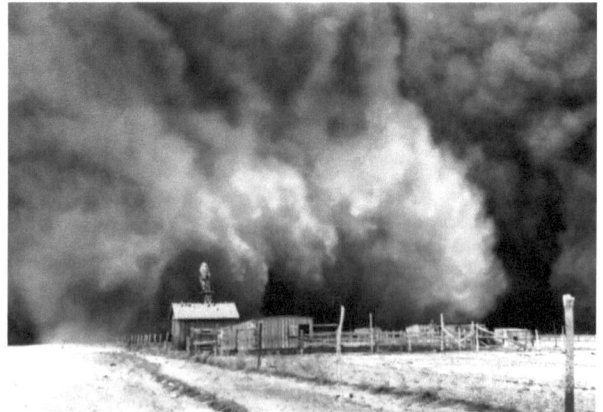

The Dust Bowl, 1935, Associated Press

Just when our country was busy overcoming these challenges and getting stronger, World War II disrupted our lives again and brought a seemingly impossible challenge for our nation to face.

The reasons World War II started are complicated. There were left over tensions from World War I, which had been over for a little more than twenty years when World War Two started. A series of invasions then caused these tensions to grow into a war involving several countries.

First, in 1935, Italy invaded Ethiopia. No one knew at the time how this would begin a series of conflicts that eventually involved nearly every country in the world. Then, Japan invaded China. Next, a man named Adolf Hitler, who had risen to power in Germany along with his ruling political party called the Third Reich, invaded Poland in 1939. This is a simplified version of the beginning of the war. There are many books that describe these events in more detail.

I've often thought about how people all around the world, everyday people like we were in Harlan, who were struggling to eat and live and get along in their communities, got caught up in a war they did not fully understand. Young men on both sides were being called from around the world to fight and risk their lives for causes they knew little about.

These three invading countries, Italy, Japan, and Germany, joined forces and became a threat to governments around the world. It is important to remember that because of WWII there were hundreds of thousands of simple lives like mine that were disrupted in order to prevent these three countries taking over other countries. It eventually became clear to all of us that they did not consider all people equal and their plan was to set up a worldwide nation, replacing all governments with their Nazi-Fascist regime.

There are thousands of books about WWII. This book is mainly my recollections as an eighteen year old. There were many American men who were given orders to bravely fight in battles around the world. These were not the orders I was given. None of us were given a choice on how we would serve our country. We all did the job we were told to do in order to win the war. It was a time of great sacrifice, cooperation, and honor. We loved our country and grew to love it more because of the great threat we faced.

On the last five pages of this book there is a timeline of events that took place from 1936 to 1945. Altogether, these events have become known as World War Two. Another way to write it is WWII. The date when I was drafted is highlighted in blue on the timeline. American boys were drafted on their eighteenth birthday and went to war.

The movie theaters seemed to be the best way to learn exactly what was going on in the war. We didn't have a TV at home. The news reel that was played before each movie helped us understand what was going on in each of the countries.

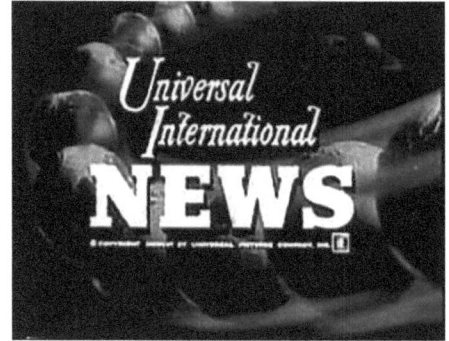

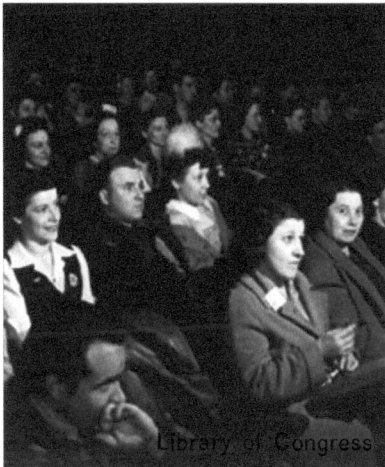

Library of Congress

It was hard to watch the clips of the violent events taking place. Most people did not have a TV and it was a new thing to see news pictures in motion.

The news about the battles and meetings among leaders and generals were also shared on the radio. People would leave their radios on all day as news reports about the battles in Europe, Africa, and the Pacific were given over the airwaves often and at random times.

The worry was constant and it took a toll on people at home. It took a toll on us in the Pacific too...always worried a bomb might land near our tent. It was a stressful time as we all did our part to keep our enemies from defeating us.

The soldiers were not the only Americans who had to stop their normal lives to fight the enemy. People who stayed in the United States did their part too. Life for them was full of writing letters, keeping rations, and working at various jobs like building tanks, ships, guns, and planes. It wasn't like more recent wars. We Americans all participated in the war effort to defeat the German, Italian, and Japanese forces and end the war. Yes, back then everyone was fully involved in the war.

We all understood, even the children, that our enemies were trying to enforce upon the whole world their Nazi, fascist ideas. Our way of life was being threatened and we knew it. We did make some mistakes along the way and I can see that now. Some Japanese Americans were forced to stay in internment camps for years. There was fear they would also become enemies of our country. It was a tremendously regrettable decision by our government to imprison so many innocent people. It was another lesson we were forced to learn.

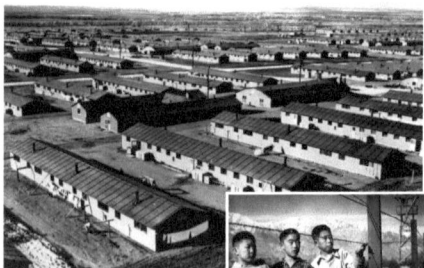

Internment Camp, Manzanar, California 1942. AP

We as a nation had never faced an enemy like this one. I believe we did the best we knew how. We were dealing with challenges that threatened our lives and culture. Our enemies were ruthless and unrelenting. There are those who criticize some decisions made by the American government but they don't fully understand the position we were forced into by our enemies. I don't think another country could have done any better in our position.

The way that Hitler was ordering his soldiers to detain and transport Jewish people to prison camps in train cars that were meant for livestock was horrifying, cruel, and evil. It terrified us to think that all of his policies and ideas could be brought to America. It is still unbelievable to me how many good, hardworking Jewish people were killed...all because of the ideas a man named Adolf Hitler.

After our goodbyes to our families and a long bus and train ride from Harlan to Chicago, it came time to learn my role in the war. As I got off the train I was told to stand in a line with the rest of the young men who said goodbye to their homes around the country that day too. When we reached the front of the line, we were told to take turns going to one of the four tables in the front of the room. We were instructed to sit with a recruiter from one of the four Armed Forces when we reached the front of the line.

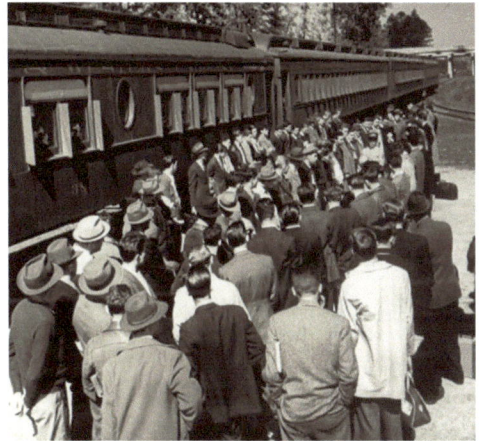

American recruits board train for transport. Library of Congress

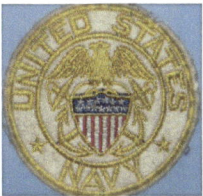

I began silently counting the men in front of me in anticipation of which of the Armed Forces I would join. I was hoping and hoping it would be the Navy. Leaning out to see down the line I counted each man. Army, Navy, Air Force, Marine, Army, Navy, Air Force, Marine, Army...then it was my turn. I was in the Navy!

Next was boot camp where we were put through intense physical training. It was during these weeks of training near Chicago that I learned it had been arranged for me to travel back to Harlan, Kentucky to give my mother blood transfusions for an illness called pernicious anemia. Pernicious anemia is a condition when a person's bone marrow does not make enough red blood cells.

The doctors said she needed three transfusions to save her life. I was a match for her blood type. I came back and forth by train from Chicago to Harlan three separate times during my boot camp before I shipped out to the war. I remember my family had to pay for the train tickets. The last goodbye was perhaps the most difficult.

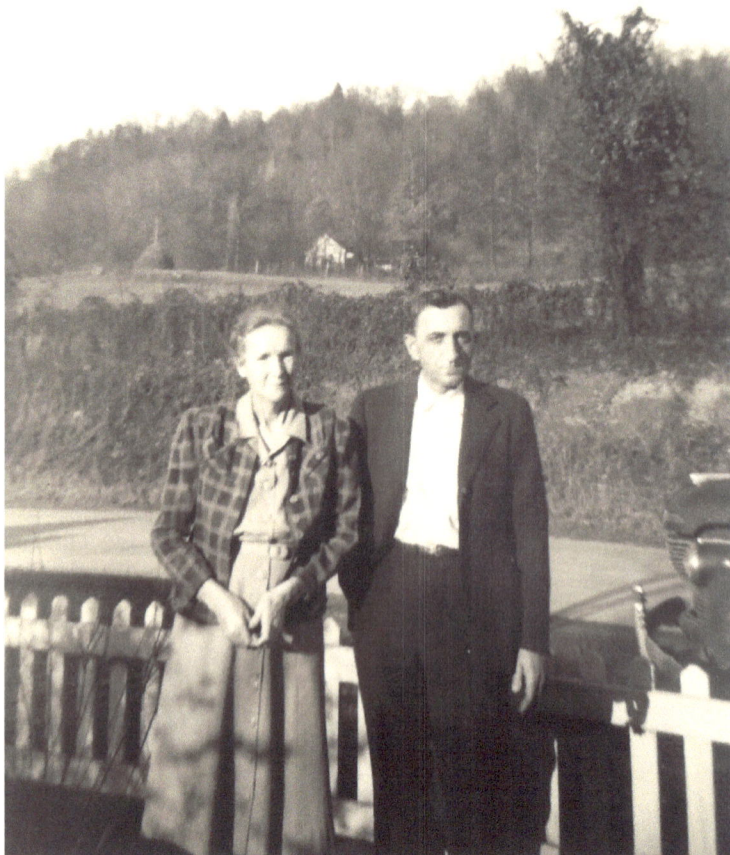

Thurman and Mary "Dinah" Brooks, parents of James E. Brooks

After several months of boot camp at the base in Great Lake Michigan, close to Chicago, I was sent to Modesto, California for additional training. At this point they would not tell us where we were going next. All they said was, "Send your blues home. You will now be issued Marine greens." These Marine greens were the uniforms I would wear for the rest of the war even though I was in the Navy.

I asked where we were going and why we needed to send our Navy uniforms home. Our superior officers said, "You will find out when you get there."

From there I was sent to San Diego, California. Again, the same answer was given to my question of where we were going, "You will find out when you get there." Everything was kept secret to prevent any information leaking to the Axis forces. We were put aboard an aircraft carrier, along with other Army and Marine troops. We still did not know where we were going or what our jobs would be.

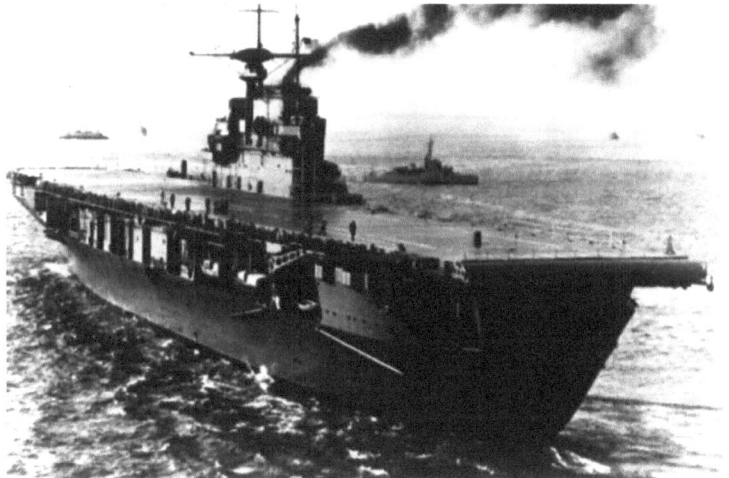

Navy Aircraft Carrier. United States Navy

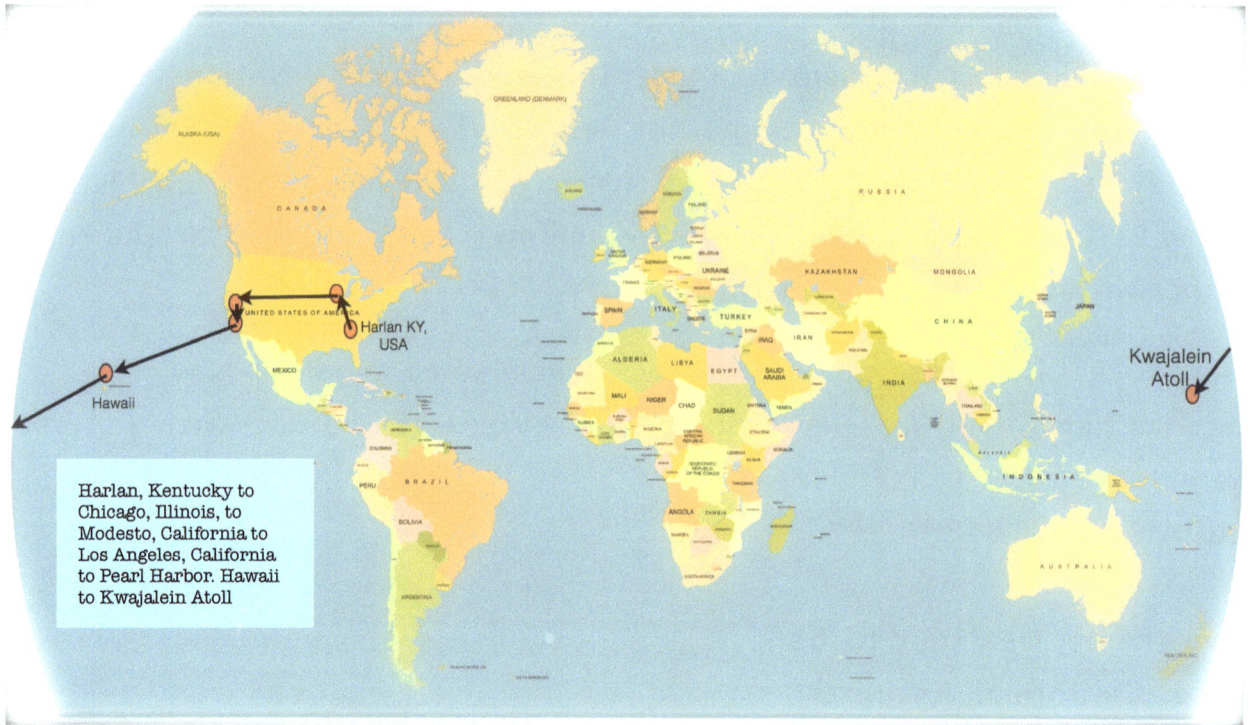

Harlan, Kentucky to
Chicago, Illinois, to
Modesto, California to
Los Angeles, California
to Pearl Harbor, Hawaii
to Kwajalein Atoll

Next, we were put ashore in Kaneohe Bay, Hawaii for further training. It is hard for me to remember now how long we were there learning various skills we would need. From Kaneohe Bay we were again loaded on an aircraft carrier for a long, seasick voyage to Kwajalein Island in the Kwajalein Atoll (pronounced Kuwajalean). An atoll is a ring-shaped group of coral and islands encircling a lagoon. Kwajalein Island was the largest of all the islands in the atoll which was also called Kwajalein. When I arrived on the island, I found out that this would be my base station where I would repair war planes flown by Allied forces in battles against the Imperial Japanese Army.

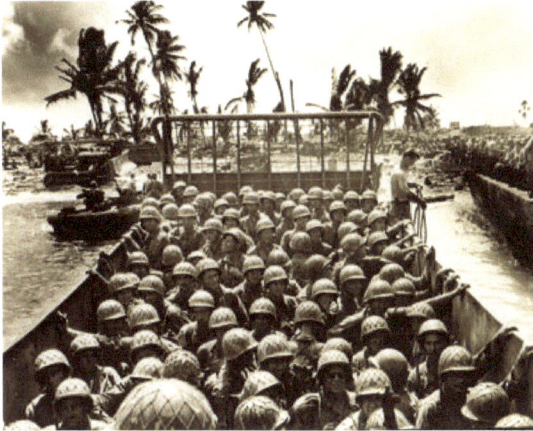

We learned that our US forces had just liberated the native people of Kwajalein from the occupation of the Imperial Japanese Army on February 9, 1944.

Troops land on Kwajalein, Associated Press

There was devastation everywhere. We were tasked with repairing war damage and cleaning up the island. We were preparing it for use as a military base in our effort to fight the Japanese. Kwajalein was the largest land mass in the Pacific used by Allied forces.

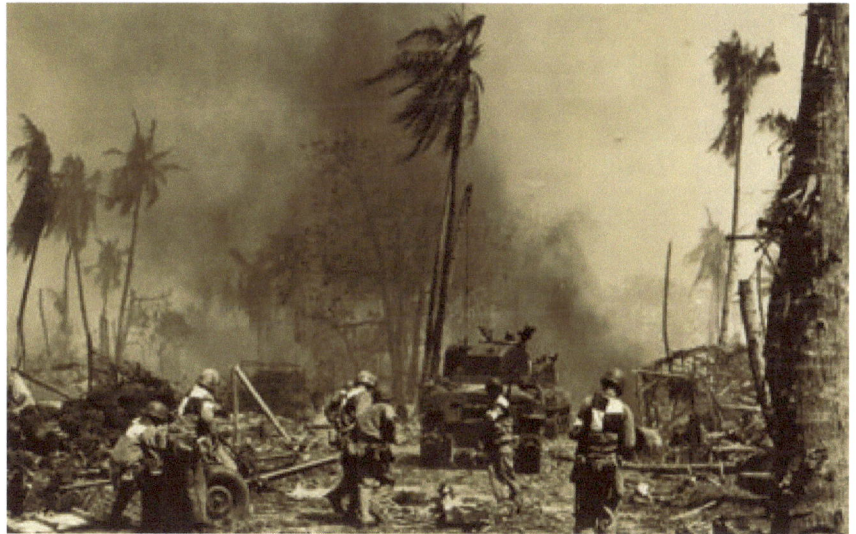

Liberation Day February 9, 1944. United States National Archives

It was a big job to prepare the whole island for use as an Allied base. We had to quickly build an airstrip where damaged American war planes could land and then takeoff after being repaired. Our job was to repair the planes that were too damaged to land on aircraft carriers out in the ocean. We also serviced planes that needed to return to other bases in the Pacific.

It is important to understand that the Americans were using Kwajalein as a stepping stone for their mission to take Tokyo, the capital city of Japan. We knew that if we were not successful, our role in the war would change. We might even become prisoners of war or be killed if we did not win the South Pacific.

I remember the slogan being used over and over again: "On to Tokyo, on to Tokyo!"

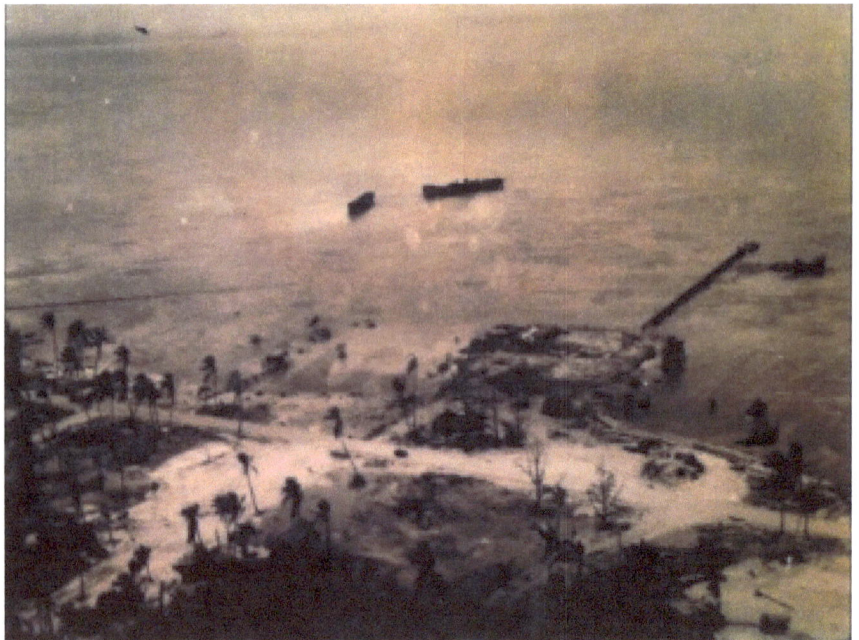

Photo, James E. Brooks

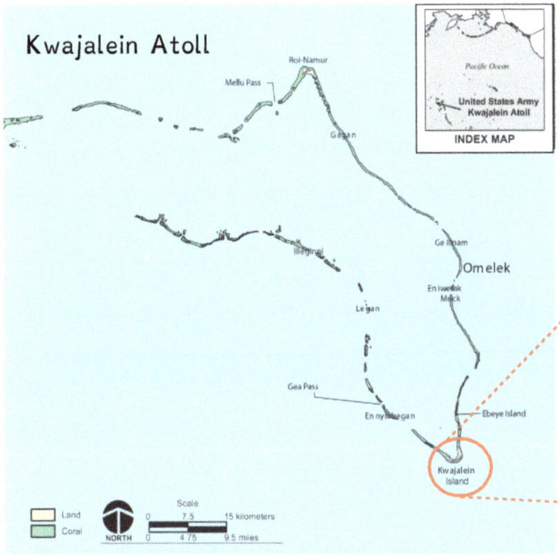

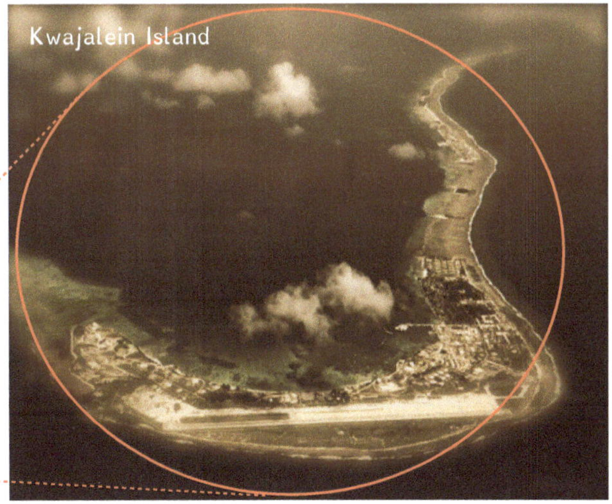

Kwajalein Atoll

INDEX MAP

United States National Archives

             I remember the islands in the Pacific
being just like stepping stones in a creek I remembered from home. Brave
pilots and soldiers fought for control of each land mass one by one.
This is a picture of Kwajalein Island taken from an airplane.

We did our best to fix the planes that were shot up by the Axis forces
in the battles, however there were some planes that could not be
repaired.

One of our jobs was to strip planes that could not be repaired of any
good parts and dump the rest into the ocean. Many people today would
not be happy that we did that, but is was something we were told to do
and had to do in the war. There was no time or space to deal with
unusable airplane parts on the island.

16

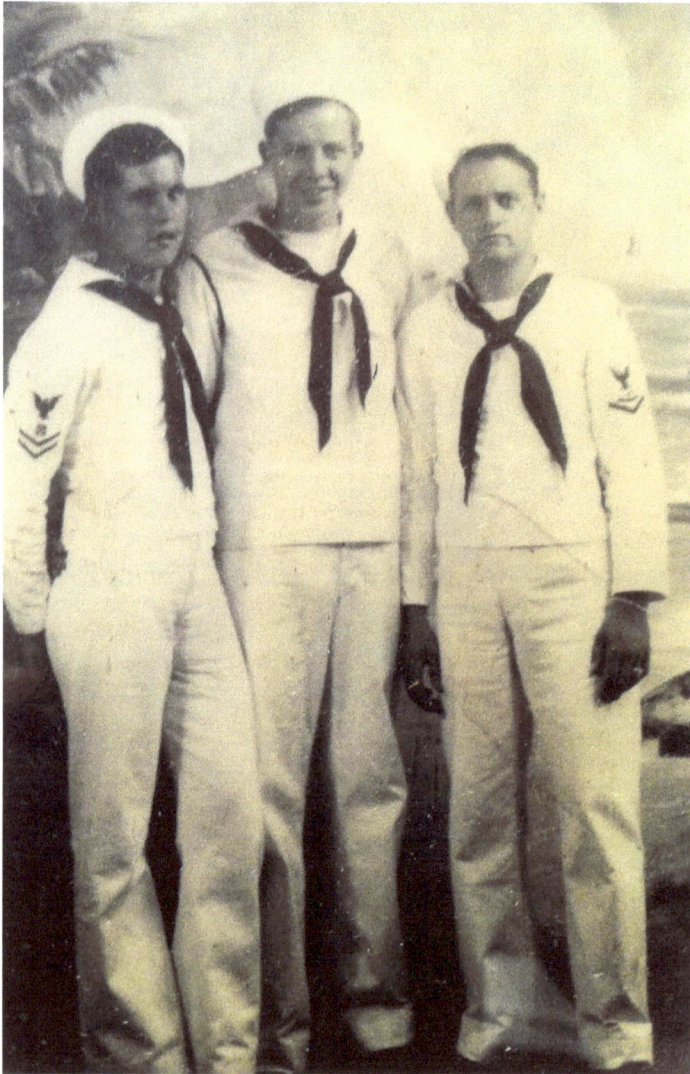

This is a photo of the soldiers I worked with and became friends with during our years on Kwajalein. From left to right are E.J. Otto, Willy, and me, James Brooks. Over the years I've forgotten Willy's last name. I wish so much I could remember it.

We lived in the same tent on Kwajalein Island for three years during the war.

In this photo, we were standing near our tent on the base. It was crowded in our tent. All of our trunks and belongings had to be kept in the tent because of the rain that frequently came. At the end of our cots we each had our own radio. We had taken them from the damaged planes that came limping back to our island. We were allowed to keep them in our tents for enjoyment after work each day. The radios did not have speakers, only headphones.

Photo, James E. Brooks

This photo shows how all the trees and dwellings on the island had been damaged by the battles before we arrived. I took this photo right after the U.S. liberation. Everything had been destroyed and we had to get it cleaned up. My first job in was to prepare the bodies of dead Japanese soldiers for burial. Remember, I was 18 years of age at the time.

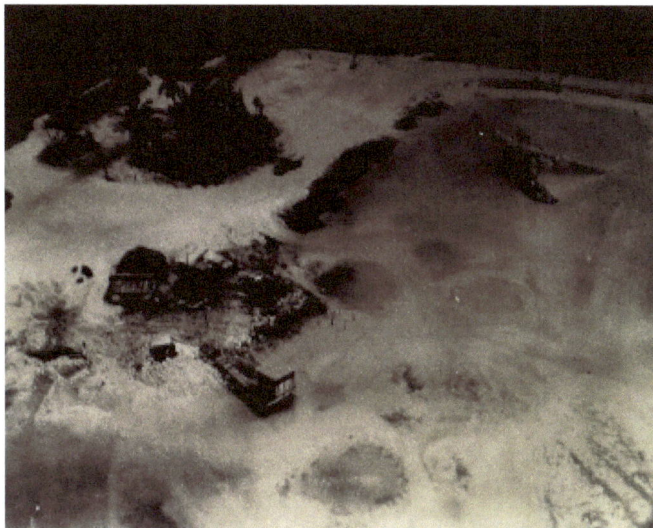

Photo, James E. Brooks

It was disturbing for me at that age to see and cope with the bodies laying everywhere on the ground. It was hard to accept what was going on. Today, it might be difficult to understand why such violence was necessary. Back then, it was clear that we had to defend ourselves against the Axis powers or our mainland would be invaded and more Americans would be killed.

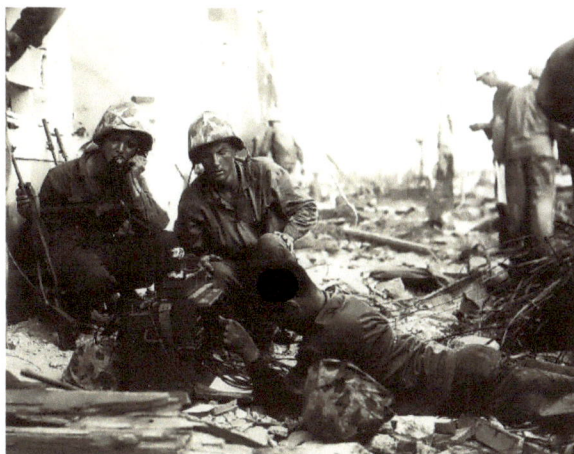

US Marine signalmen setting up a command post in the streets of Roi-Namur, Kwajalein, Marshall Islands, 1 Feb 1944. United States National Archives

At first, I couldn't sleep at night, always seeing in my mind and dreaming about the disturbing things happening around me. Sleeping in tents and outside in the middle of the South Pacific sure was hard on all of us. However, we knew that fighting back was necessary, especially after what they did to us at Pearl Harbor three years before we landed on Kwajalein.

Before the Imperial Japanese Army attacked the United States at the American military base in Pearl Harbor, Americans believed it was best to stay out of the war.

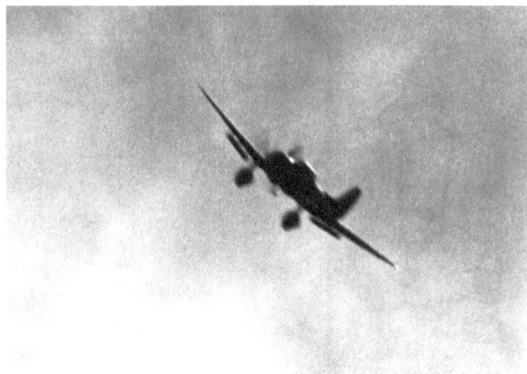

AP Photo

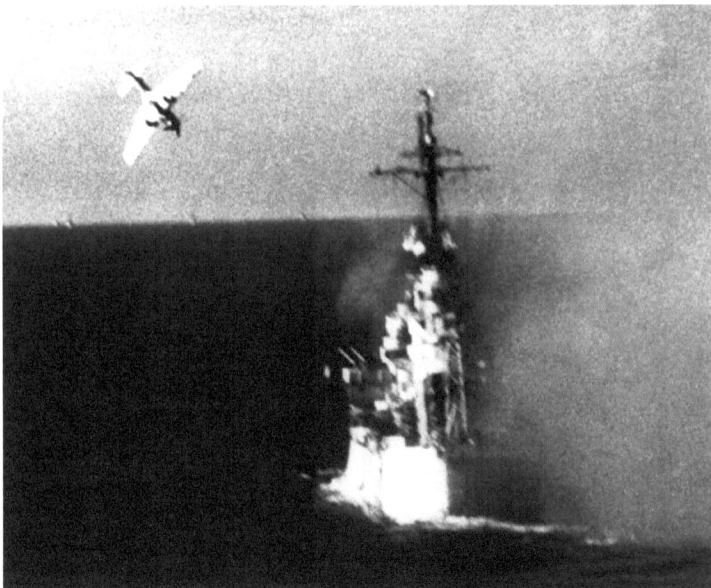

AP Photo

This opinion, which was held by most of us in America, was called non-interventionism.

The attack on the American Military Base at Pearl Harbor by the Imperial Japanese war planes killed 2,402 Americans and wounded another 1,282. When this happened, many Americans changed their minds about how we should be involved in the war.

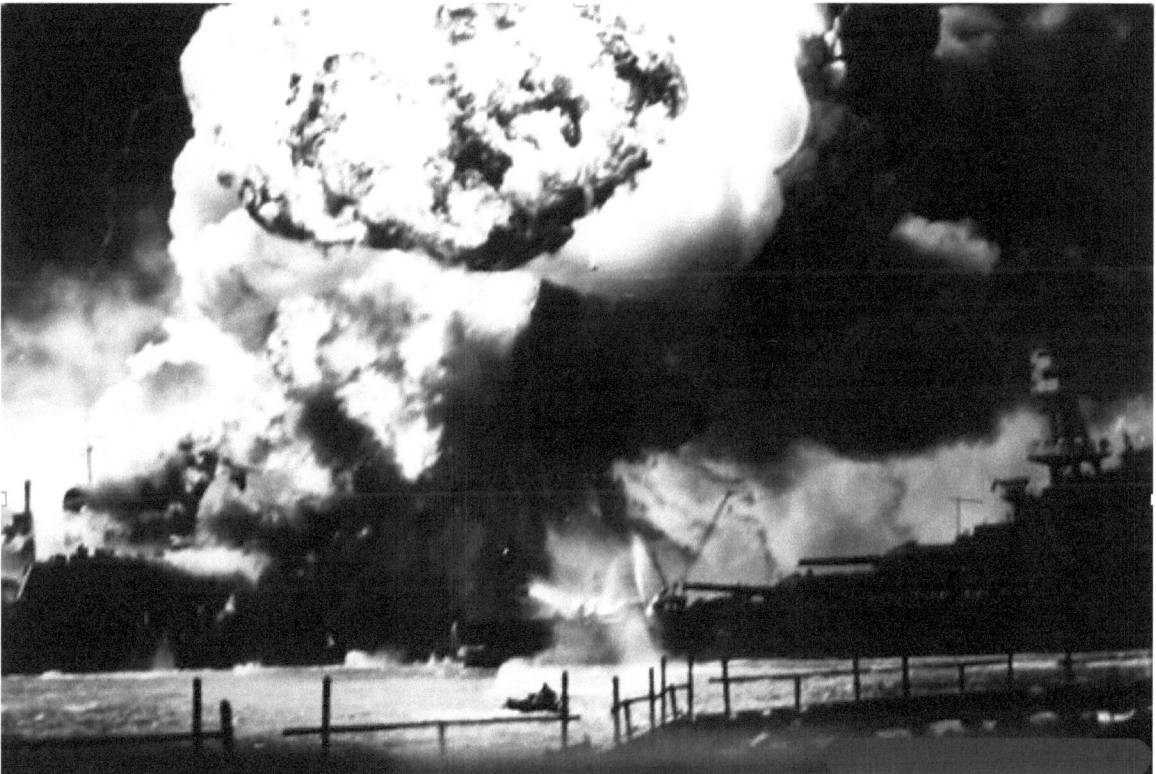

Pearl Harbor
December 7, 1941
United States National Archives

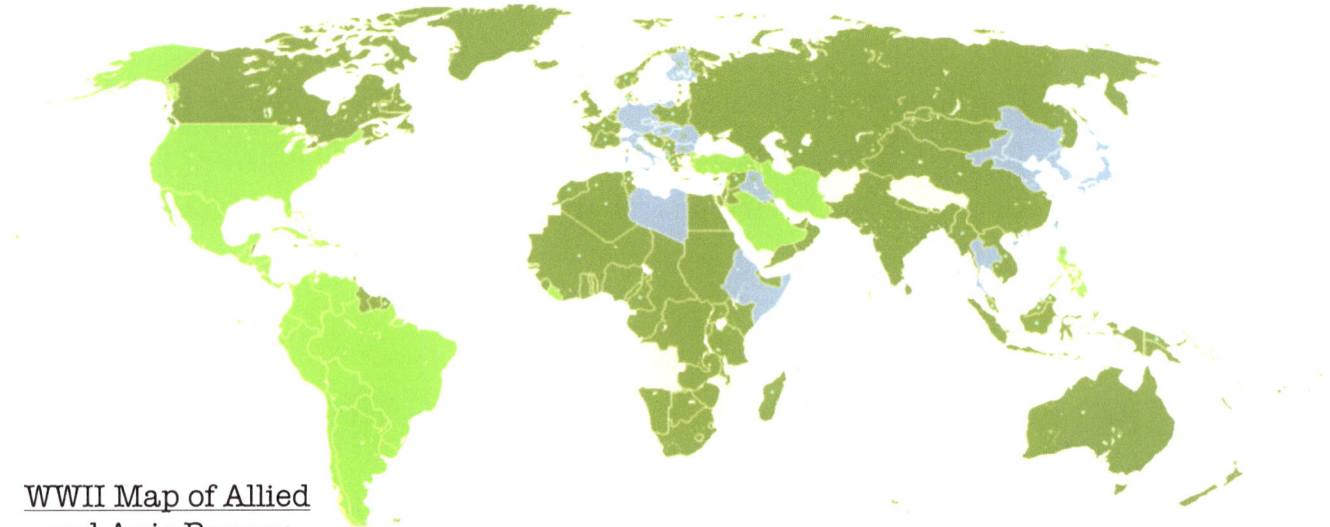

WWII Map of Allied
and Axis Powers

Allied Powers
Axis entering after the Attack on Pearl Harbor
Axis Powers
Neutral Powers

More and more Americans began to believe that the continental United States would be invaded and conquered by the joint forces of Germany, Italy, and Japan if we did not join the war effort against them. The three countries of Germany, Italy, and Japan became known as the Axis powers. These powers continually lied to other world leaders about how many countries they planned to take over. It was hard to determine whether or not the Axis would ever stop invading other countries. The countries that decided to fight against the Axis were jointly named the Allied powers or the Allies. There were some countries that chose not to fight at all. These were called the neutral countries.

On the island we listened to the radio to learn some of what was happening across the world. It was difficult to understand all the details from just radio broadcasts. There were no cell phones or computers because none of these things had been invented of course.

Again, our main focus was straightening up the island after all the battles between Japanese and American troops. Then it was on to the work of repairing planes for the rest of the war years. I felt every plane that came in for repair was mine to taxi. Taxi means to drive a plane along a tarmac. I rushed out to each one, traded places with the exhausted pilot, drove them onto the tarmac, and parked them in order of repair priority. They started calling me hot pilot as a nickname because I would stop what I was doing and run to meet the planes. We all got a laugh about that.

I enjoyed repairing all the engines, wings, and propellers. Oh, but my favorite thing to do was taxi the planes and diagnose the problems with each plane. This is a photo of me taxiing an SBD (Scout Bomber Douglas).

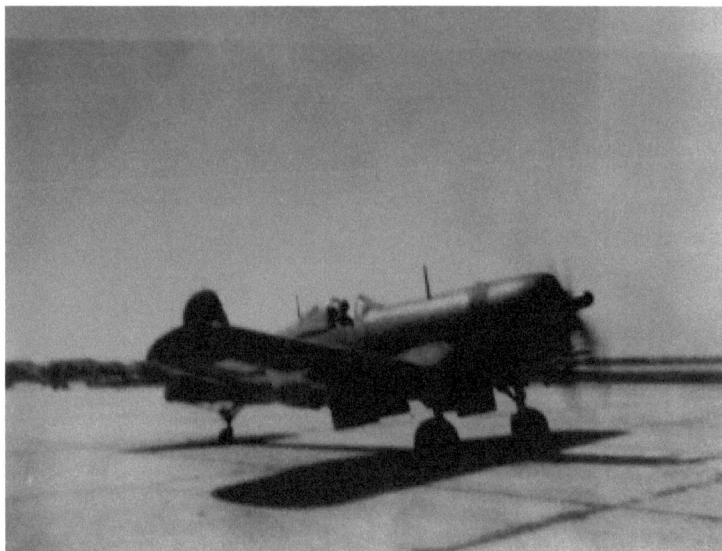

Photo, James E. Brooks

When a pilot landed he would speak to me about the problems the plane was having. He would describe the sounds and knocks the engine was making and we would try to diagnose and fix each issue. Sometimes a pilot and I would go up in his plane to get a better picture of a problem. This helped us more quickly identify what was wrong and get a plane flying at it's best for action. I took this photo during one of these trips up with the pilots.

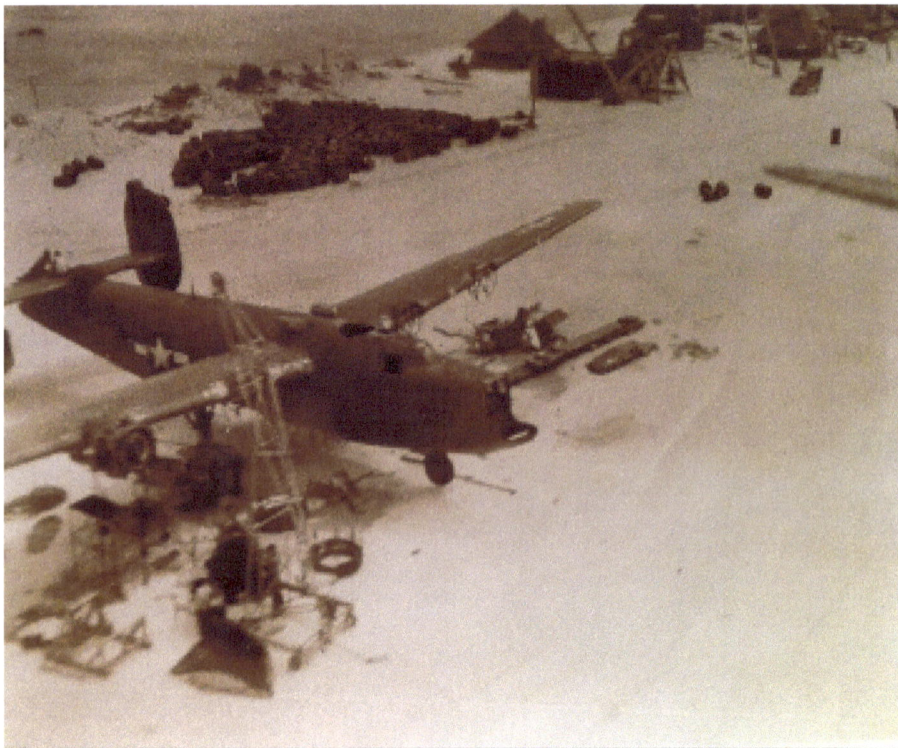

Photo, James E. Brooks

We often found that it was easier to check on what work needed to be done as a plane was in flight. Even after our repairs, we would have to go back up again and listen to the engine so that the pilot would point out things we may have missed.

Oh, the planes would come in really shot up. Most of the planes we repaired were terribly damaged and destroyed from the battles with Japanese fighter pilots.

You see, the Japanese planes were much faster than our planes at the beginning of the war. Then, toward the end of the war, our second run of fighter planes were much improved and much more successful in battle.

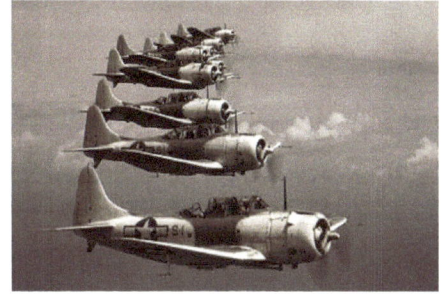

AP Photos

The Americans back home designed and manufactured faster planes quickly.

We dumped so many of our destroyed planes off the coast at the beginning of the war, but later in the war our pilots did better in battle and we were able to repair these less damaged planes. We dumped fewer and fewer planes as the war went on. Our main job was to get them back into the air. This is a photo of some of my friends working on plans to repair damaged planes.

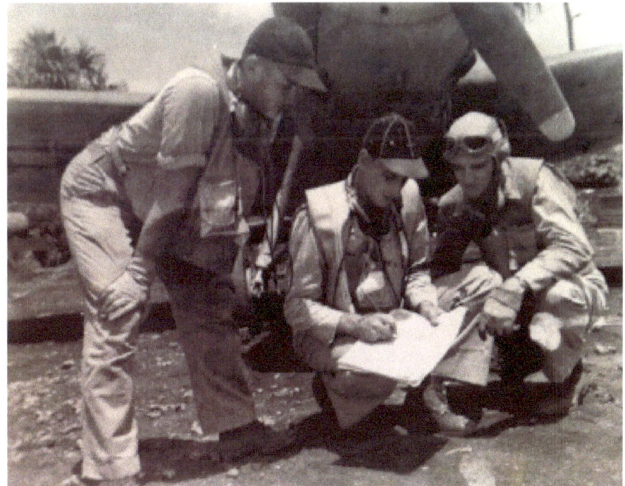

Photo, James E. Brooks

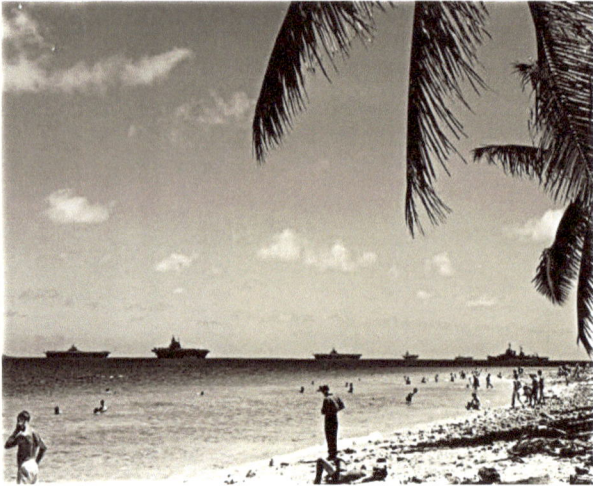

My tent was right on the water. I could hear the waves all night. It was nice to hear the tide come in and out.

United States National Archives

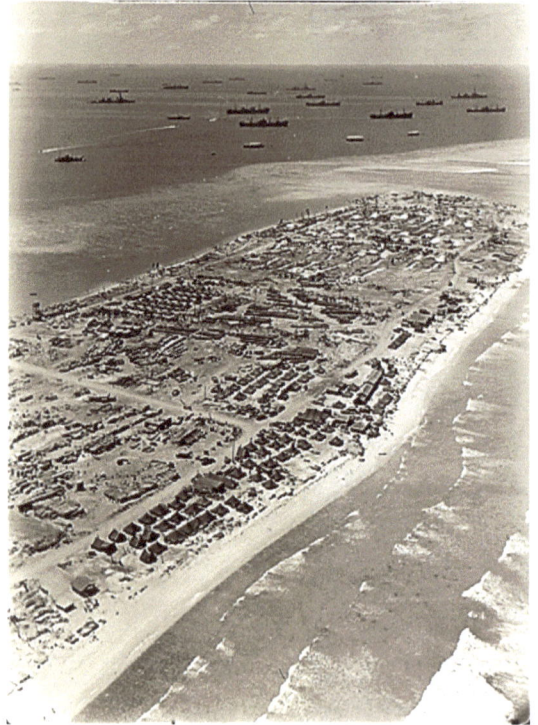

Kwajalein of the Marshall Islands becoming an American advance supply base.
United States National Archives

On Friday afternoons my friends would swim out past a underwater wall way out off the beach and spear lobsters. I wasn't a good swimmer so I didn't venture out into the waves with them. They would bring the lobster to me on the beach as they caught it. We would then build a fire right on the beach and boil the lobster in a large barrel of water.

Everybody would eat as much as they wanted. We always had tables set up where we would prepare the lobster and then we'd sit together in the sand and eat. Oh, there was nothing but sand everywhere it seemed. It was a kind of a party for a time and oh, the lobster tasted so good.

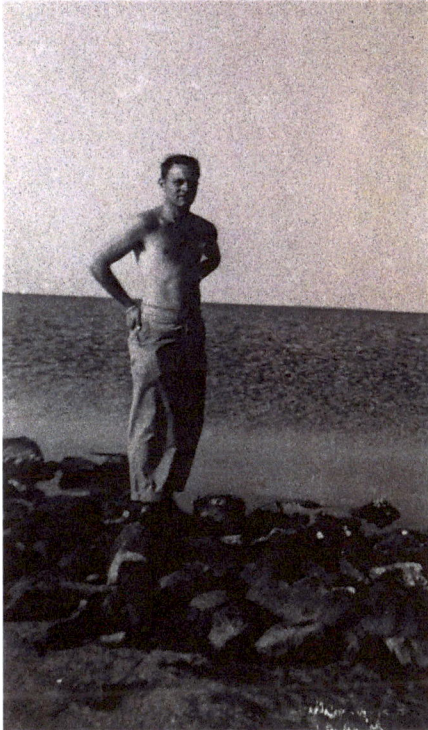
Photo, James E. Brooks

The party would have to be over before dark. You see, we couldn't afford to have a fire going because the enemy would surely spot the light from the fire and drop bombs in the night when we couldn't see their planes to shoot them down.

In fact, one night, when I was on patrol, I got myself into a bit of trouble. This was a time in my life when I really enjoyed cigars. It was way after dark I was smoking a cigar as I took my turn on patrol walking the beach. My senior officer saw me from far away and reprimanded me there on the beach.

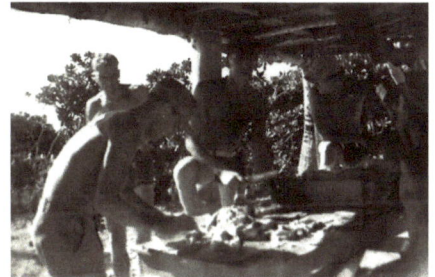
Photo, Marine Bombing Squadron 613 Paul Yanacek

"Brooks, do you realize what you're doing?"
"Yes sir, I'm on guard duty," I replied.
"Do you realize the danger the light on the end of your cigar is bringing?"

I told him I didn't realize I was doing any harm and I would be sure not to do it again. Even the small light of a cigar would have been visible to enemy planes.

From time to time different flights would land on Kwajalein to refuel for long trips, and occasionally there would be movie stars on the flights. They would get off the plane and walk around the island a bit. Glenn Miller, a famous singer, and his band came to the island once. I didn't get to shake his hand but I could see that he was friendly. His plane went missing from enemy fire shortly after that and it was never found. It was another sad loss.

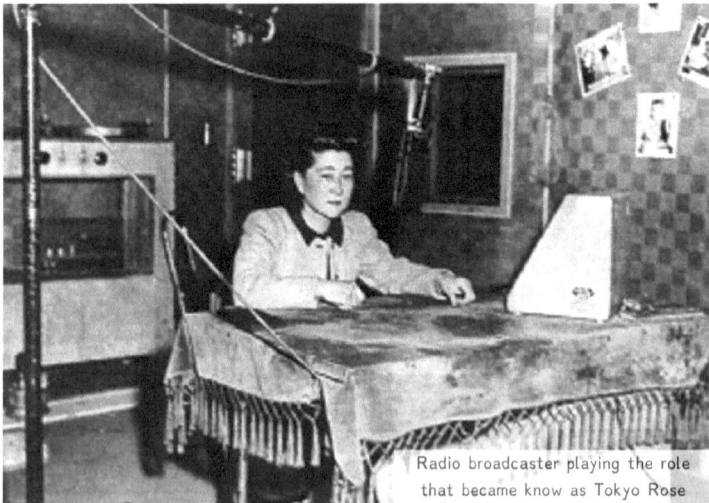

Radio broadcaster playing the role that became know as Tokyo Rose

Every night as we fell asleep, we listened to the only radio channel we could get on our radios. It was broadcast out of the capital of Japan, Tokyo. American soldiers had invented the name Tokyo Rose for the host of the show. There we were in the dark, each with our own radio set up on crates and trunks at the end of our cots, with our earphones on trying hard to sleep. Of course, we could not see what the host of the show looked like. I was surprised to see this picture of Tokyo Rose after the war was over.

This radio show was the only way we could listen to music from home. Tokyo Rose played music we desperately wanted to hear. She played all our favorite songs but was emotionally cruel to us in between the songs. The Imperial Japanese government forced her to say things that would upset us and make us homesick.

We couldn't help but listen to these radio shows because we all longed for home and the songs were like a bit of home each night. I remember the songs "Shoo Shoo Baby" by the Andrew Sisters, "Moonlight Serenade" by Glenn Miller, and "Wonder When my Baby's Coming Home" by Helen O'Connell with Jimmy Dorsey and his Orchestra. Tokyo Rose played songs by Glenn Miller and Frank Sinatra that were all "heart-breakin" kinda music.

I learned later that there were actually several women who were forced into this role of broadcasting propaganda to the Allied forces as a way to weaken the resolve of our service men and women. Later, they were given pardons for the role they played in the war. I felt sorry for them and how they were mistreated by their leaders.

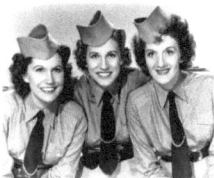

The Andrew Sisters

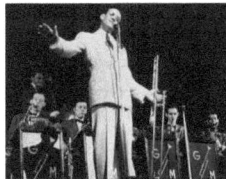

Glenn Miller

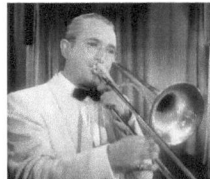

Tommy Dorsey

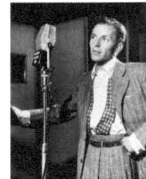

Frank Sinatra

We laid on our cots with our earphones on every night after the officer called lights out. We got use to the broadcasts and the hurt from what she said finally went away some; we got more comfortable with her cruel teasing and we could enjoy the life of the American music she was playing.

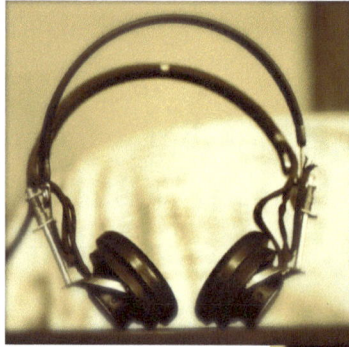

Headphones and Radio taken from a Destroyed WWII Plane

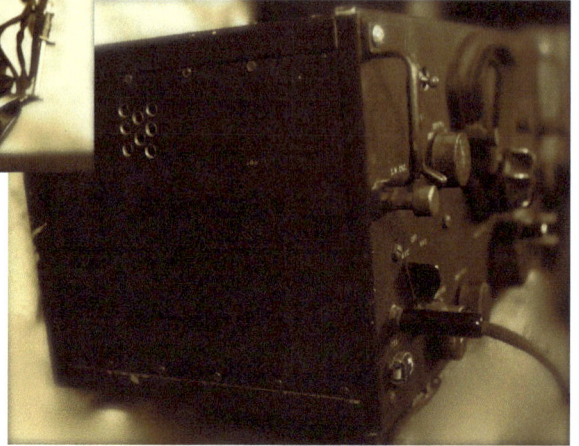

In between songs she would say things like, "Your girlfriends back home need you, dont you miss them? You should go home. You will never win this war. You can't win this war, we are stronger. The Japanese are going to take over the United States"

There we were, many of us just 18 years old, laying there hiding our tears in the dark, trying to be brave, scared to death of what could ultimately happen to us, our families, and our world. Yet, as a homesick teenager you're just not going to turn off the songs of Glenn Miller, Tommy Dorsey, Frank Sinatra, the Andrew Sisters, and Bing Crosby because it was too nice to hear a little something from home. We had seen so much gruesome death and we needed a little bit of home.

Church services were given each Sunday in the Chapel. Many soldiers attended and we sang hymns and listened to sermons given by the chaplain who was stationed there with us or other visiting chaplains. I remember a tragic incident where five chaplains were killed along with their entire ship's crew when a kamikaze plane sunk their ship right off our coast. It was especially sad for us.

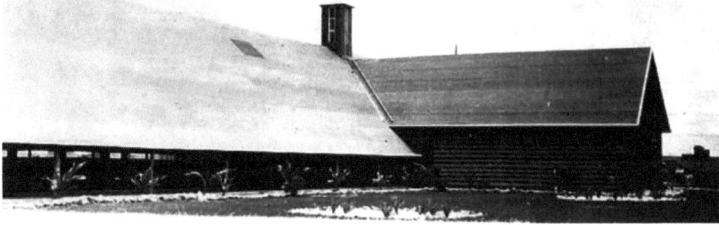

Kwajalein Chapel, U.S. Marine Corps (Courtesy of William A. Kehr) vmb613.com

These days people don't like to talk about some of these things that happened to us all. It is the truth and it's important to remember.

Once, for example, many years later when I was sharing my memories with a large group of high school students, someone didn't like how we had to dump some of the wrecked planes into the ocean. He asked me not to share this part of the story. He didn't understand that we were trying to win a war that we didn't start and we needed room to work on the planes that could still be repaired. It wouldn't be done the same way today, but I hear that the dumped planes now make for good underwater habitat for coral and sea life.

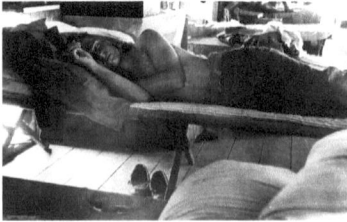

Everyday was hard work. The heat was especially grueling some days.

Usually we would go the beach and relax a little on Saturdays. It was only 100 yards or so to the beach from our tents. We would swap information from our letters from home. It was always interesting to see who had the biggest tale to tell from the letters they received.

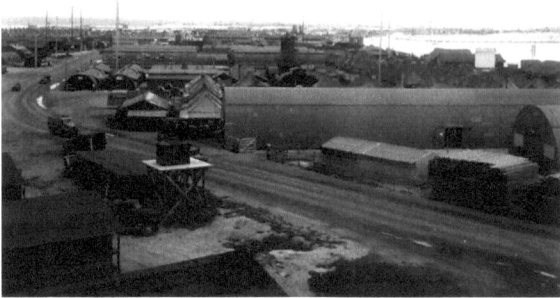
Kwajalein Atoll Base 1945 U.S. Marine Corps. (Courtesy of Diane Hindy) vmb613.com

I didn't have a girlfriend at the time to get a letter from but many did. Mother and Dad always wrote, bringing me up to date on all the news from home in Harlan County.

We would see a movie or two after time on the beach on Saturdays. The movies were shown near our mess hall that was another 100 yards away. There was an old movie projector with reels that projected the movie on a large screen.

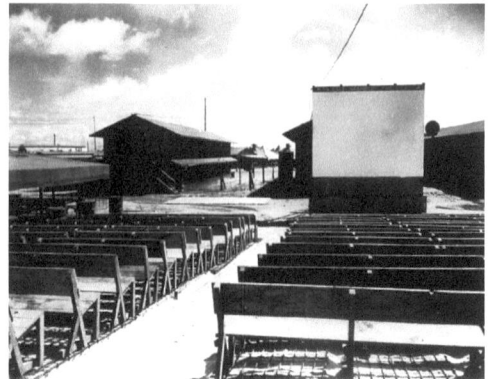
Kwajalein, U.S. Marine Corps
(Courtesy of William A. Kehr) vmb613.com

There were Army, Navy, Marine, and Air Force service men and women...all of us there together. Some were there permanently while others were just moving through. It was quite a place with so much going on.

It was the largest island in the South Pacific which is really amazing to me still.

The native Kwajalein people spoke English and we worked together often, helping each other with food and relaxing together with movies and music from time to time. I remember seeing some westerns on the movie screen. Once, the USO gang with Bob Hope came to Kwajalein. It was a big surprise because we were in no way expecting them. The show had some seriousness and then of course lots of comedy from Bob Hope.

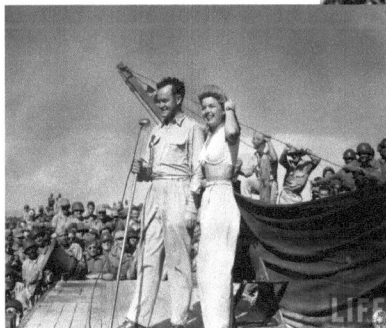

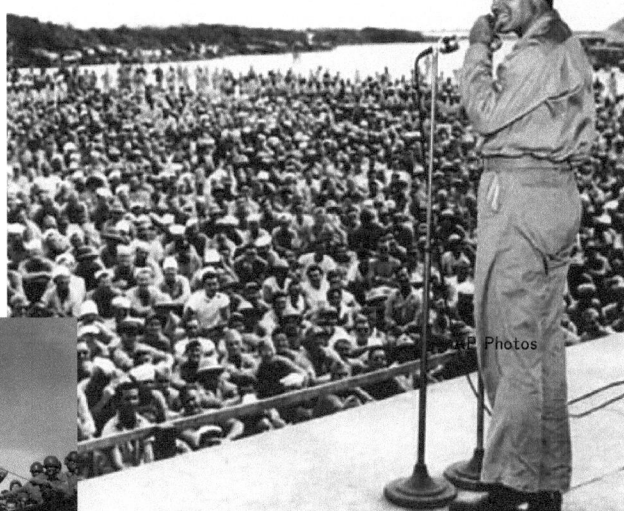

There were challenges of all kinds. The war caused tremendous economic hardships. Americans had to ration their sugar, hosiery, tires, gas, oil, cheese, cars and many other goods. These items were needed in the war effort, therefore each person was allowed a certain amount of these important products. This is a picture of a ration book for fuel oil. Each ration stamp could be used to purchase a specific amount of the product.

United States National Archives

Each person was given a certain number of these stamps per month from May of 1942 until December of 1945. Even children had ration books. Once a person had used his or her ration of sugar, for example, they had to wait until the next month to get more.

There were many Americans who changed jobs and moved to another part of the country to help build ships, weapons, and uniforms. Lives everywhere were disrupted in an effort to fight the Axis Forces and the Nazi-Fascist nation they were planning to create.

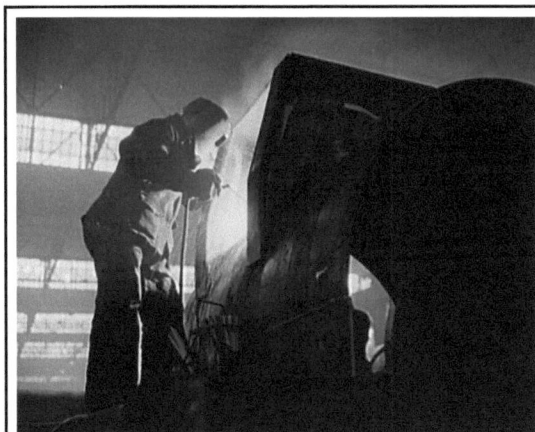

"Liberty" ships. Welding was more important than ever before in shipbuilding, saving time, weight and steel. All parts were prefabricated in this huge plant which formerly turned out freight train cars. Baltimore, Maryland. Library of Congress

I have been blessed to live a long time. I'm 89 years old now. My memories are not staying with me as well as they have in the past and I know I repeat myself sometimes. As I think back about the war, the main thing that comes to mind now is how many millions of families lost their loved ones because of what only a few bad men started.

I took the photo on the next page near the end of the war. I took it, along with all my other pictures, with a camera I borrowed from a friend.

I wanted a picture of how the people who were native to Kwajalein could climb the trees to pick coconuts. They would call it skinning up the trees. None of us could ever master this, and oh how we tried. It was just like walking for them, getting up there in no time. We became friends with them over the months we were there.

I took this photo near sunset one night. We had a beautiful sunset nearly every night. I couldn't wait to show it to my family when got I home. I really wanted my mother and older sisters, Maxine and Ercel, to see how beautiful the island was after our clean up right before the end of the war. The war effort was going well in Europe and we all knew the war could be over soon.

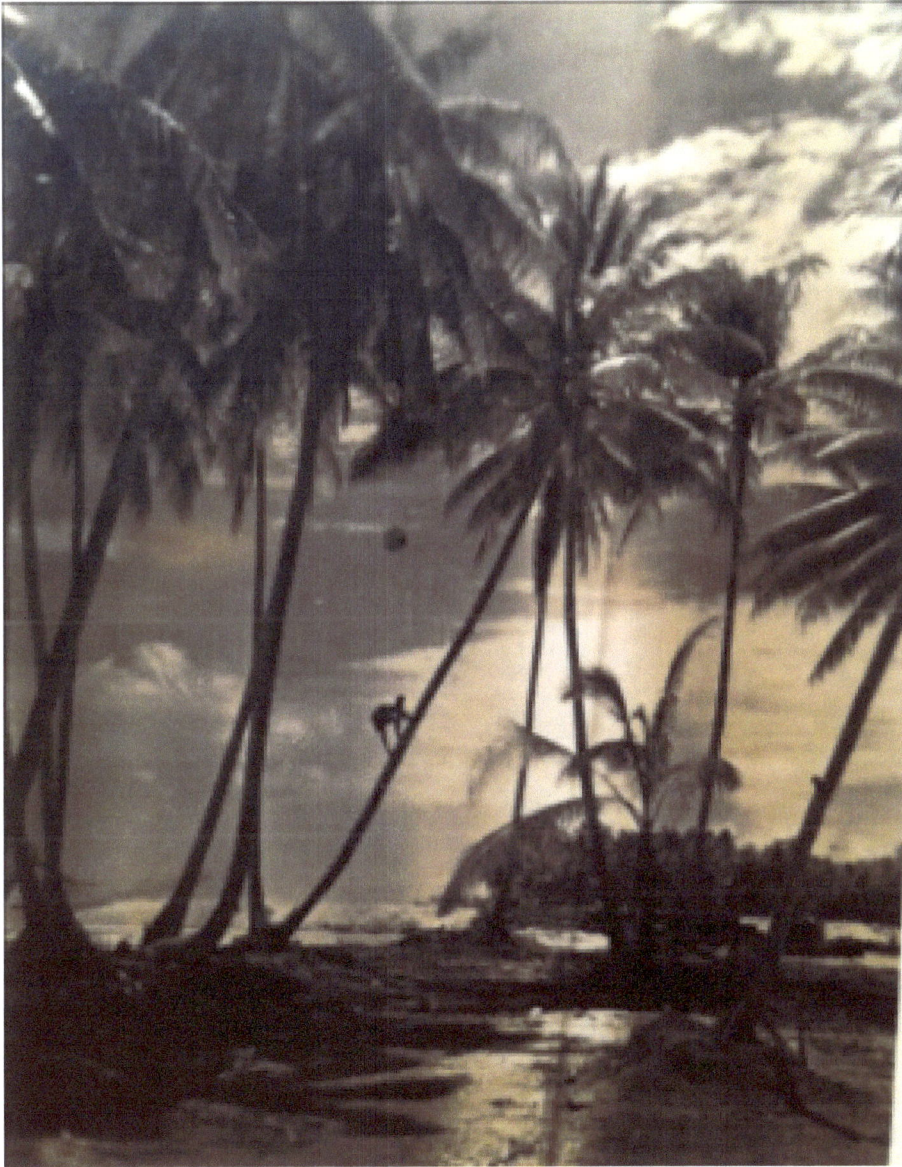

Photo, James E. Brooks

Then, the day the whole world was waiting for came, finally we received word that the war was over! On September 2, 1945, the Japanese signed a surrender treaty.

Japanese Foreign Minister Mamoru Shigemitsu came aboard the battleship USS Missouri and made the agreement with US General Douglas MacArthur. A massive formation of American fighter planes, some we likely repaired, flew over the USS Missouri Battle Ship as the agreement was made. This treaty was significant because it marked the end of the war in all theaters, Europe, Asia and the South Pacific. This day was called V-J Day which means Victory in Japan. We all celebrated on Kwajalein. We hollered and whooped all day and night when we heard the news!

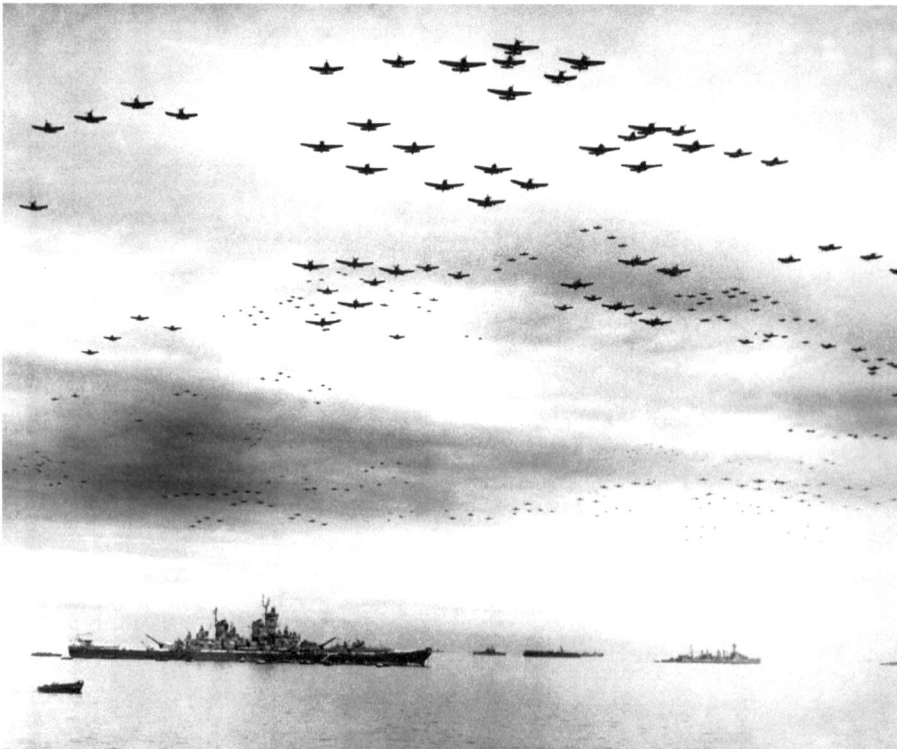

USS Missouri Battle Ship, V-J DayUnited States National Archives

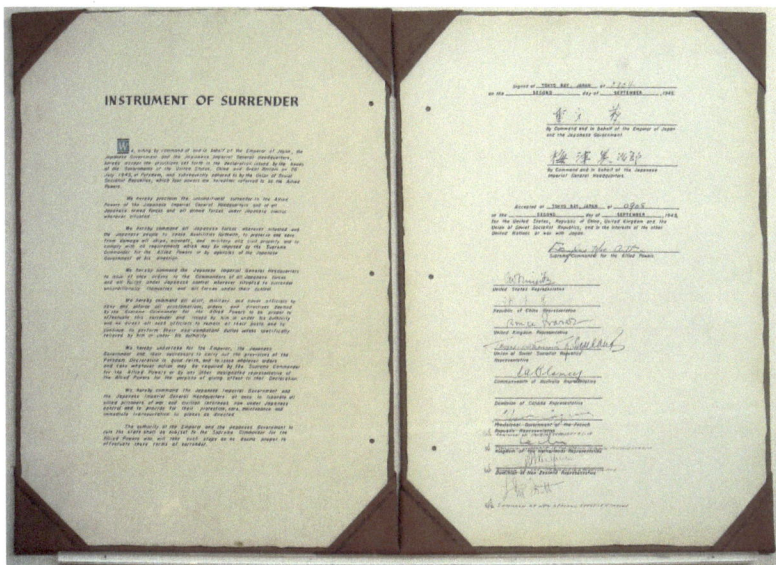

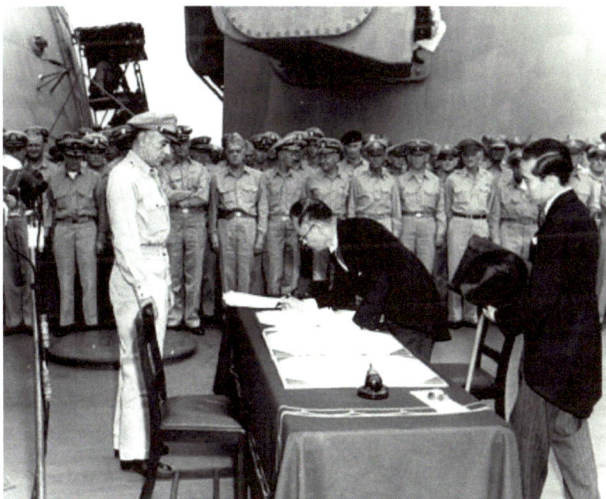

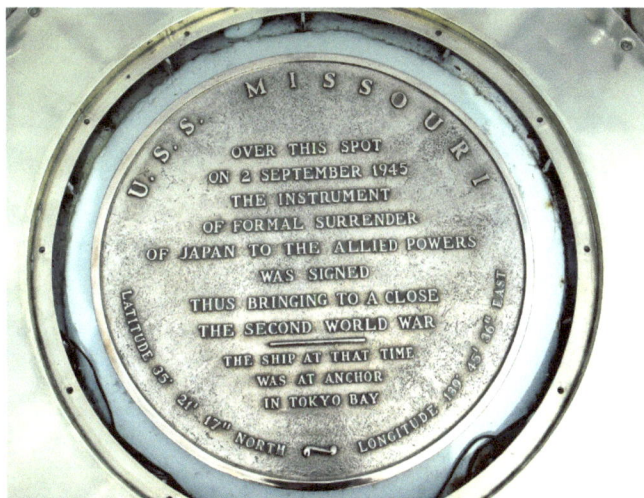

United States National Archives

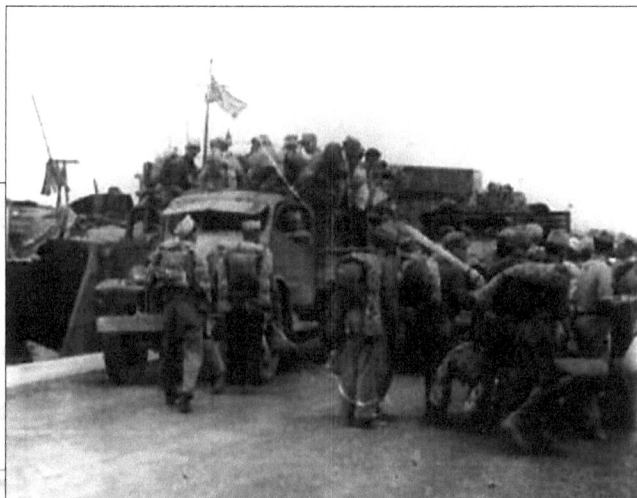

Packing to leave Kwajalein. vmb613.com

We packed all the tools and equipment in just a few days. After our long seasick ship ride, we arrived Hawaii. We each hugged and shook hands with one another as we got off the ship. I had worked with these men, side by side, for three years. There were many soldiers already there in Hawaii ready to get home. Eventually, on various days, we were shipped to California.

Once I arrived in California, I went with my friend William to his home where his parents were overjoyed to see him finally home, safe and sound. After all these years I dont remember his last name. I never saw him again. I sure would like to find him again and talk about our memories of WWII on Kwajalein. I do remember his father was an MGM movie director.

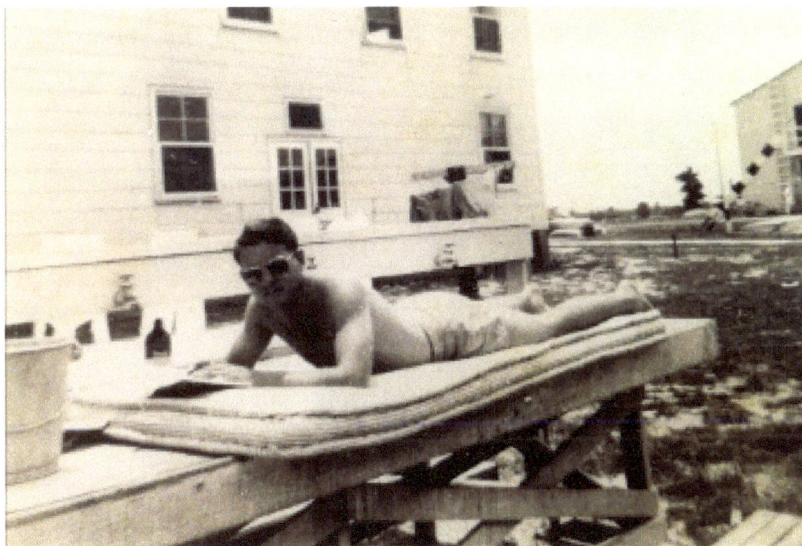

Photo, James E. Brooks

Next on my journey home to Harlan, Kentucky, was a long cross-country train ride to Memphis, Tennessee, where I stayed on the Navy military base a few days awaiting discharge papers to return home.

This is a picture of me sunnin' in Memphis by the barracks right after the end of the war. I was looking so forward to seeing my family and friends.

So many families were devastated as Marine, Navy, Army, and Air Force soldiers were killed. These men and women made great sacrifices for the liberty we have today. I still believe that if it hadn't been for the men and women back at home, who worked hard to manufacture the war planes and equipment, the outcome of the war may have been very different. We all needed each other for victory.

It is estimated that 60 million people were killed worldwide in WWII. There were many battles over islands in the South Pacific. There was Tarawa, Saipan, Iwo Jima, and more. The battle for Iwo Jima lasted 36 days. There are many heroic stories to read about these battles.

The Japanese, along with the other Axis forces, were eventually found guilty of many war crimes during World War II, including the killing of up to 20 million Chinese people. We lost an estimated 100,000 Americans in battles with Japanese forces. The Japanese policy called "Kill All, Burn All, and Loot All" and their use of biological weapons and torture led to many Japanese leaders being executed and imprisoned after the war. It is difficult to speak of now; we can forgive but not forget the lessons we learned. We are good friends with the country of Japan today. We must remember how the deceptions of a few corrupt leaders led to such harm so that we don't make the same mistakes again as a civilization. I often wonder if the citizens of the Axis countries knew of the true intentions of their leaders before the war started.

As I look back 70 years, I'm happy to be here and turn another page. A lot of water and daylight has come and gone. I'm glad to put on paper the memories I still have. I hope people who read my words better understand what happened to boys like me in those war years. I hope that they'll never have to go through a war like the one we had to go through in the 1940s. It was hard for all of us to keep our heads above water for a while because of the toll the war took. There were so many friends and acquaintances of mine who were killed or wounded. Lives were changed forever.

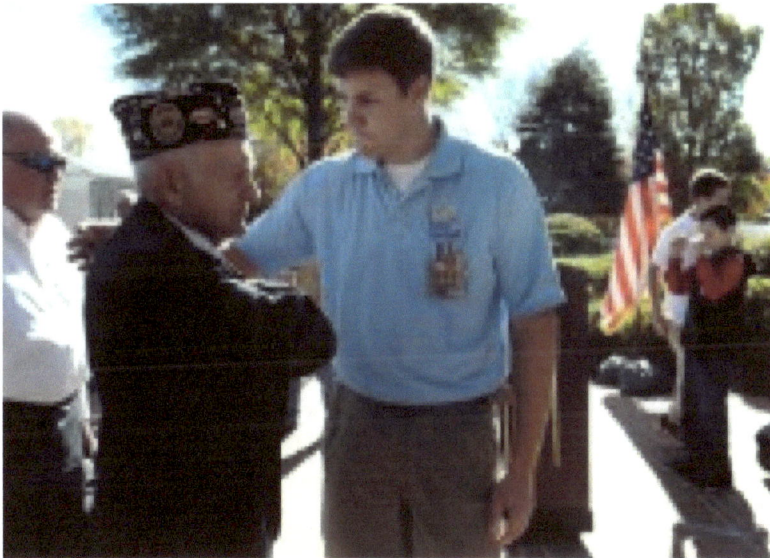

World War II Flight of Honor Day, Washington, DC photo, James E. Brooks

I'm a charter member of the World War II Flight of Honor now. We all feel good about the work we did. I know I can put my hand on those planes and say, I did good work. The reason the war had to be fought was because of the Axis powers who wanted to conquer the world. It sure was an awful hornet's nest that started small and was terribly hard to put out.

After receiving my papers I thumbed my way to Knoxville, something that is too dangerous to do today. I was trying to save my money. In Knoxville I decided to use the money the Navy had provided me to buy a bus ticket the rest of the way home. I made a phone call at the bus stop in Tazwell, Tennessee to let my family know I would be arriving in a few hours.

My dad met me at the bus station in Harlan. I remember my dad hugging me for a long time and saying, "I'm glad to see you son." On our ride home, we talked about my long adventure to Kentucky from the Pacific. For many days to come we spoke of my time in the war. He listened to the details about airplane repairs and the cleaning of Ebeye, Enewetak, and Kwajalein.

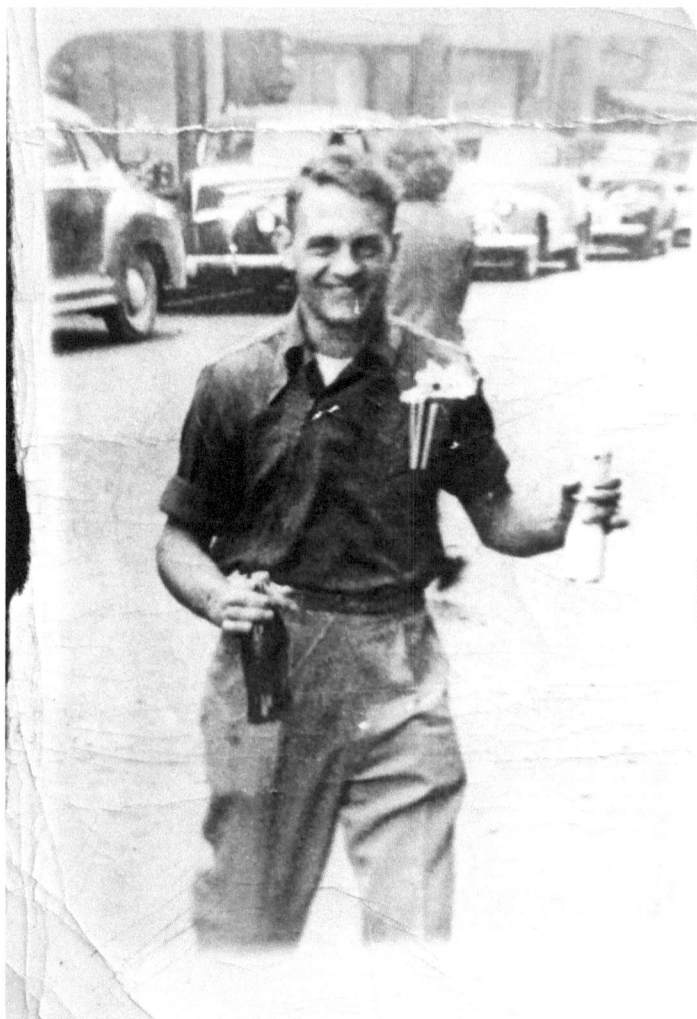

Photo, James E. Brooks

As I arrived home I found my mother just where I knew she would be, in her kitchen cooking meals for the coal miners. I remember she was so glad to see me. She hugged me with her apron still on. I picked her up off her feet with my hug. She was a quiet woman but this day she screamed, "Jimmy! Jimmy!" as I spun her around and around. We all laughed and laughed.

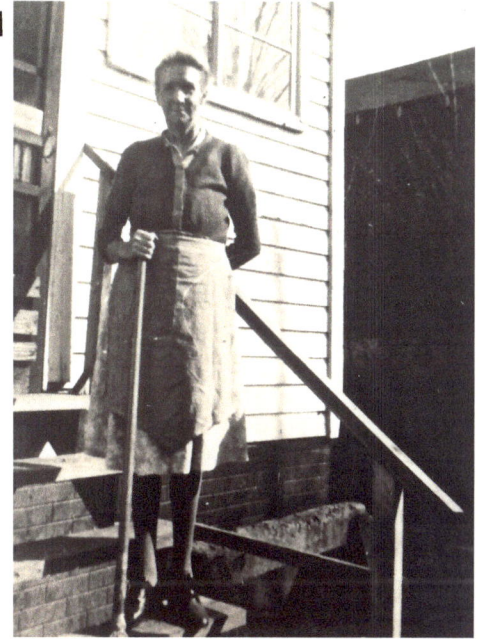

Dinah Winchester Brooks, mother of James E. Brooks

I told her about the things I had seen. I knew she would be interested in hearing about the flowers on all the islands. I told her about the coconut trees, how beautiful Kwajalein was, and about the kindness of the native people there.

As I look back, I am sure the native Kwajalein people were happy we freed them from the Imperial Japanese forces. We had good relationships with them.

I was happy to see my sisters, Maxine and Ercel. There were hugs all around. We sat down to my favorite meal my mother cooked. It was fried chicken and dumplins, all homemade of course! Oh, and biscuits, gravy, ham, soup beans, corn bread, and apple pie. We lived a simple life, with few belongings but we always had plenty of Mother's good food.

It had been about three years since I had seen my family when I got home from the war. It was good to catch up with family members and friends. I had a cousin who had been a prisoner of war in German-occupied Russia for six months during the war. He was home too. We compared our memories and kept in touch often. His name is Glenn Brooks. He was 15 when he volunteered to enter the war.

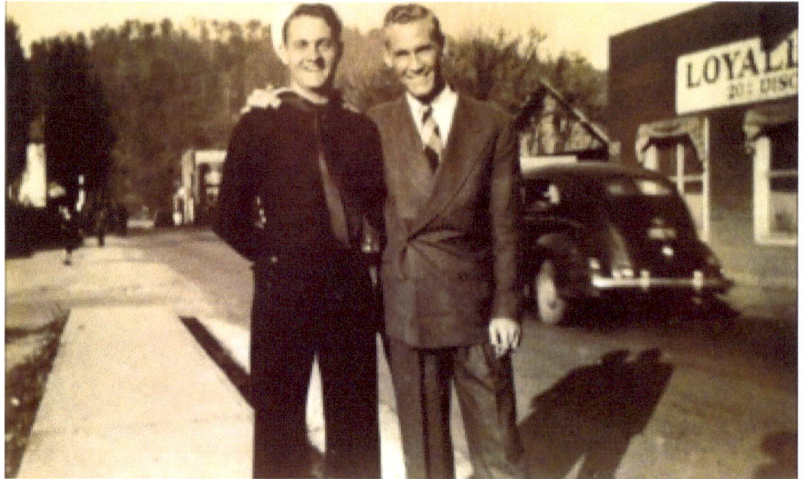

James E. Brooks and Glenn Brooks, 1945.   Photo, James E. Brooks

The recruiter told him, "Sorry, you have to be 16 to volunteer."

Glenn replied as a spirited 15 year-old would, "Well, I can't help that."

They decided to pass him through anyway. He eventually became a Bird Colonel, which means he was the highest ranking colonel and right under Brigadier General.

Glenn told me how it was a 16 year old girl who helped him escape the POW (prisoner of war) camp where he was being held. Hundreds of American prisoners of war died in these prison camps because of the poor treatment, lack of adequate food and healthcare, and sometimes torture. Glenn was so grateful for the girl who risked her life to help him escape. He wished he had a way to connect with her to thank her, but he was never able to.

There were many sons and fathers who did not return home. Many were buried at sea, wrapped in an American flag and slid down a board into the ocean water in the Atlantic or the Pacific. So many of our soldiers died in prisoner of war camps after they were captured by our enemies.

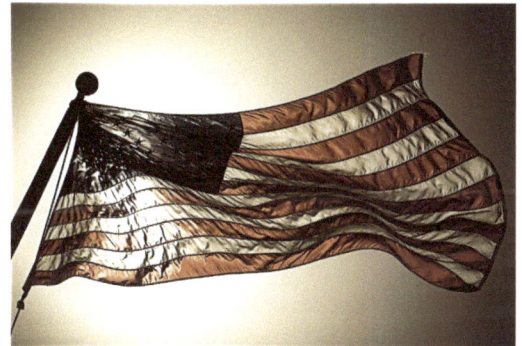

Creative Commons, CC

All over the world, our men and boys were lost because Hitler, Mussolini, and Hito wanted to be rulers of the world. I think about it often and it seems to me that the worst of it started because Hitler hated the Jews so much. He believed some people were more worthy than others to have health, liberty, and happiness. It is still hard to make sense of it, maybe because it doesn't make sense. Hitler gained more and more power through his persuasive speeches. There was much talk about his skill as an orator for years to come.

I couldn't help but think about this often, maybe because I worked for a Jewish family a few years after my return home. I spent a great deal of time with them, the Steinbergs. I learned retail management and a good work ethic from being employed at their business. Proper tailoring, style, and financial management were skills I learned from Mrs. Steinberg and her family at The Quality Shop in Harlan. I learned so much from them. After becoming friends with them, it bothered me more and more to know what had happened to their family members and all the Jewish people in the war. How could anyone hate an entire people group? The war had caused them so much worry and devastation. The world did not know of the exact number of deaths or the unspeakable brutality the Nazis caused the Jewish people until after the war was over. During the war the Steinbergs brought many of their family members from Europe to live in Harlan

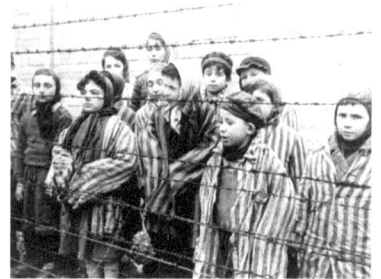

Young survivors just before being freed from the Auschwitz Concentration Camp. Public Domain.

to escape harm's way. Perhaps the lessons about never allowing another Holocaust are most important. This is another topic worth more focus than I have room for here. There are many good resources for learning from this horrific human tragedy.

There will never be another war exactly like WWII because of our new technology, diplomacy, and communication but there are still dangers and new threats. We don't want our children to live through a time where families' lives are disrupted, businesses are destroyed, and children and high school students cannot attend school.

Oh, as I think back the women and older men went through hardships too, building tanks, planes, and ships to help in the war effort. Coburn and Cora Howard, who would later become my mother-in-law and father-in-law, moved from their home in Harlan to Michigan to help build B-24 bombers during the war.

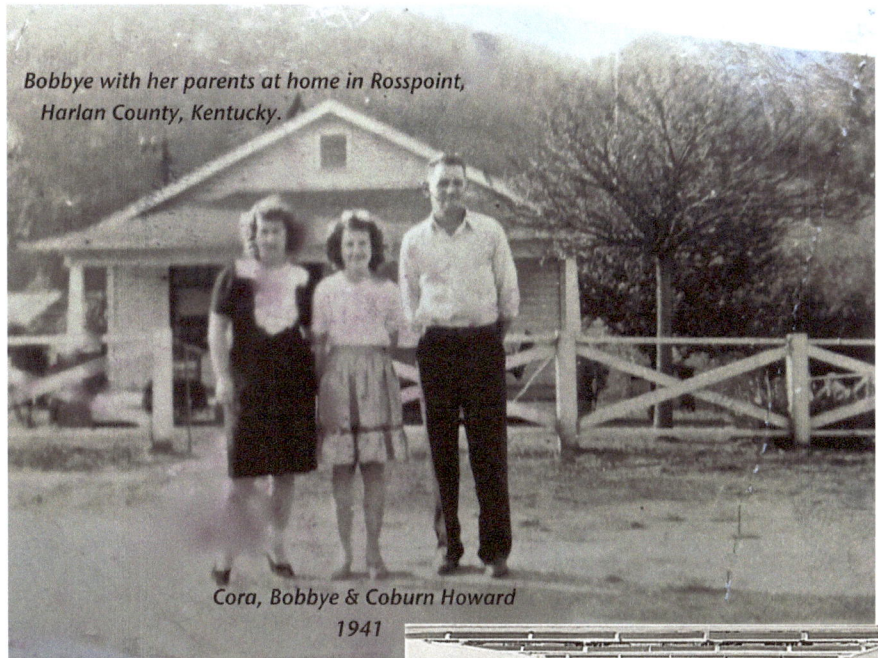

Bobbye with her parents at home in Rosspoint, Harlan County, Kentucky.

Cora, Bobbye & Coburn Howard
1941

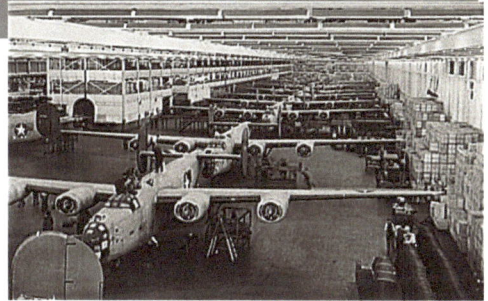

B-24s under construction at Willow Run Michigan.
Library of Congress.

Their daughter and my future wife, Bobbye Howard, stayed with her grandparents when her parents moved to Michigan. Bobbye is seven years younger than I am and she was attending Loyal High School at the time of my return from the war. I had missed the last two years of high school so I picked up again as a junior when I got home. When I finished high school, I was several years older than most of my classmates.

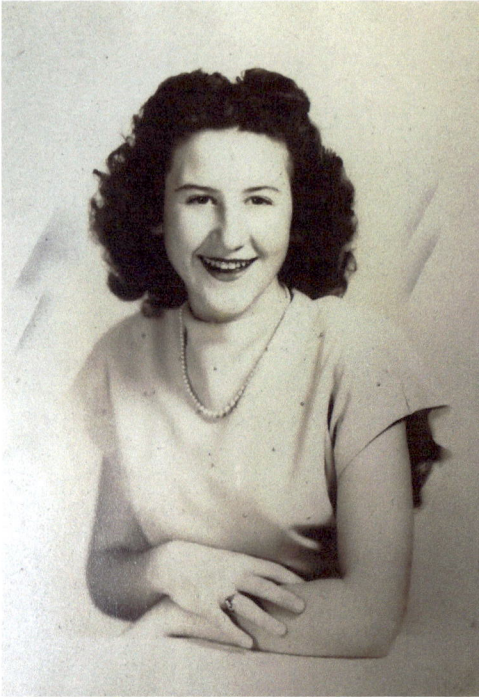
Bobbye Brooks

Before reenrolling in school, I first looked for a job and ended up doing odd jobs around town, one of which was delivering flowers for the local florist. One day my task was to bring flowers to Loyal High School. I planned to attend there the following school year. That was the day I first met Bobbye. She was working in the school office helping out. The flowers I was delivering were for a school banquet later that evening. I gave her the flowers and we had a little visit.

As I was leaving the office I turned around and looked back at her and said to myself, "That's the girl I'm gonna marry someday." I called her again and again until she agreed to go on a date with me.

We had many happy times in high school with our friends. We were in the school choir together and we really enjoyed our trip to Silver Springs, Florida in 1949.

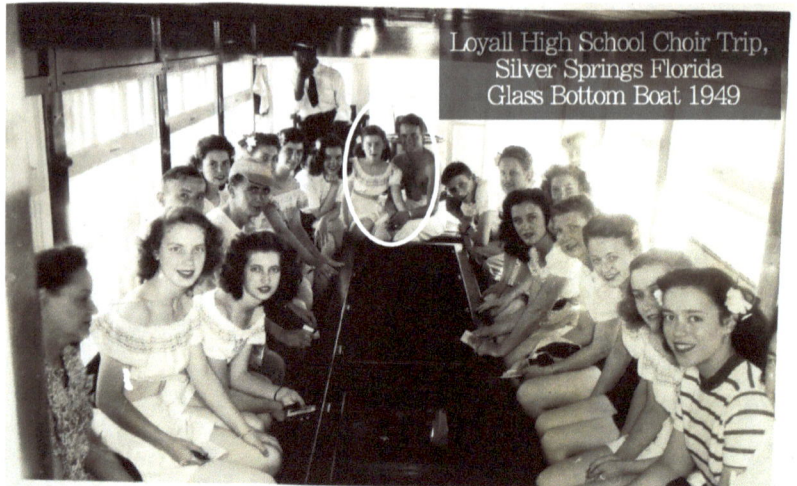
Loyall High School Choir Trip, Silver Springs Florida Glass Bottom Boat 1949

Bobbye was lovely and kind to everyone she met. I did indeed marry her in 1949 on Christmas Eve at the church parson's house. We went to Evansville, Indiana for our honeymoon.

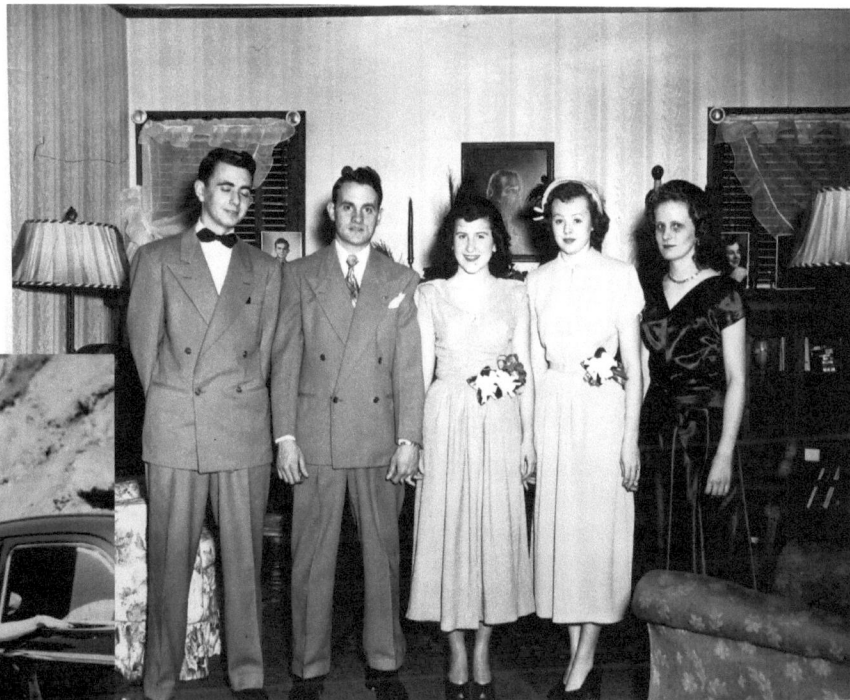

Our Wedding Day

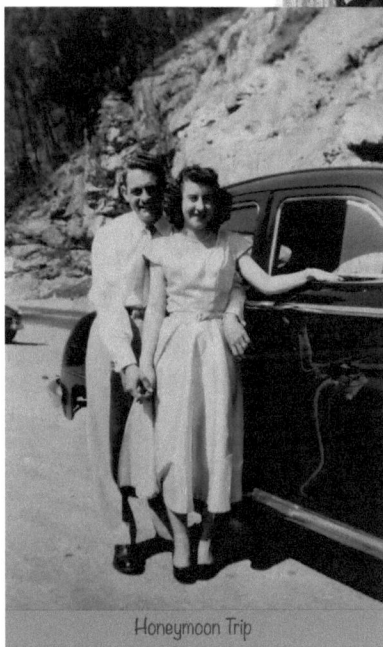

Honeymoon Trip

Oh, we went so many places with our friends, concerts, beach trips, lakes, and dances (jitterbug was the dance we loved to do).

We had our favorite places, country clubs and dance halls. Owners and managers would invite the two of us

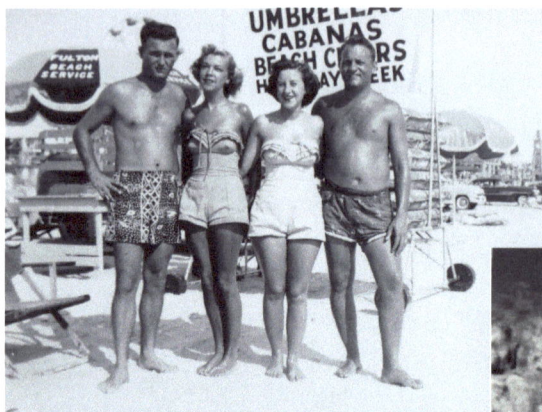

Fun times with friends at the beach

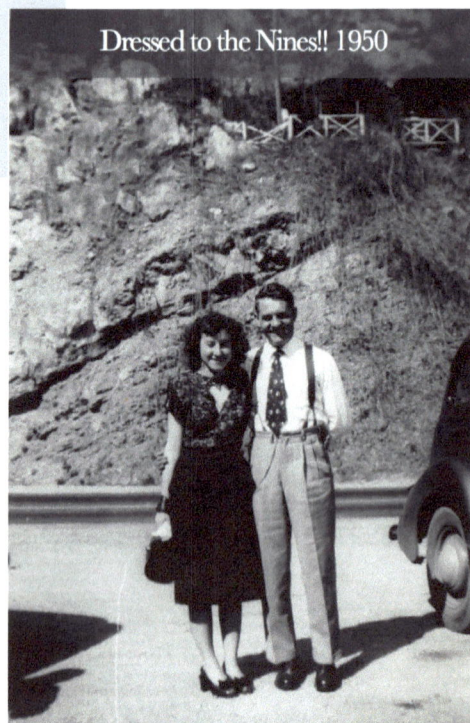

Dressed to the Nines!! 1950

to come and dance for them. People would watch us and then join in. There was a place called the Dairy Bar in Baxter where we especially loved to go and dance with friends till really late in the evening, 11 P.M. or so. They were good times and happy memories!

My dear mother eventually passed away from pernicious anemia and my father too, from a condition called black lung which is caused by breathing coal dust in the mines. They had also done there part to bring happy days to our country. The coal industry provided most of the energy to build what our nation needed to win the war.

After working odd jobs around Harlan for a while, I got a job as a manager of a gas station at the Harlan Motor Company, where my engine training from the Navy came in handy. Later, I was hired at the Quality Shop Clothing Store owned by the Steinberg family. This is where I got my start in merchandising. Bobbye worked at the Cumberland Valley Music Company in downtown Harlan. Back then, when customers would come into the store to buy music, they could go into one of many booths and listen to the record before they bought it.

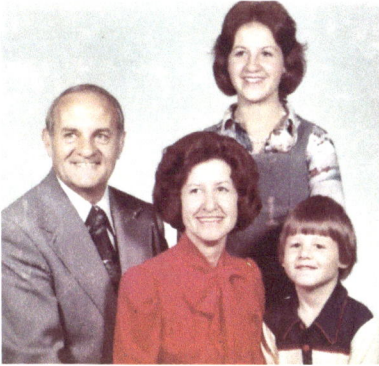

James and Bobbye Brooks with their children Jennifer and Preston, 1974

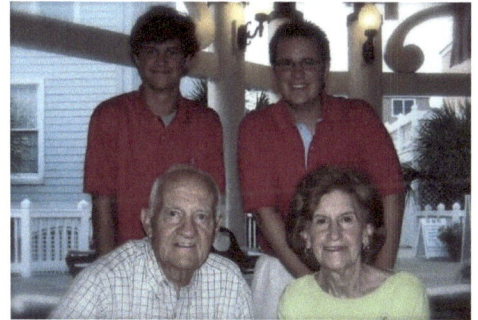

James and Bobbye Brooks with their grandchildren John Michael Griffith (top left) and Brian Griffith (top right)

After ten years of marriage, our daughter Jennifer was born in 1959. She made us so happy always sayin', "Daddy, I wanna sleep in your'alls bed tonight." Preston, our son, was born ten years later in 1969. We were so proud when he was born. Jennifer thought he was her baby doll. Now we have two grandsons and an extended family we love so much!

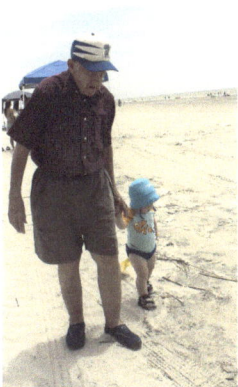

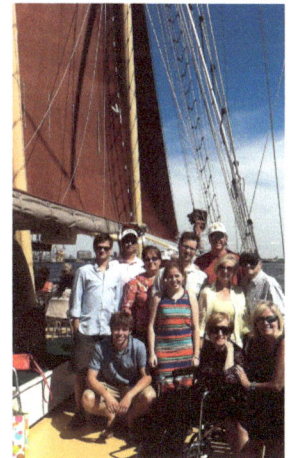

We have had a full, happy life in a world much better than it would have been without the hard work and sacrifice of so many people during WWII. I hope younger people realize this, and I hope we have learned enough to prevent an enemy like we had in WWII from rising to power again.

We have come a long way in developing healthy relations with the countries we were enemies with then. The United States has become good friends with the countries of Italy, Germany, and Japan.

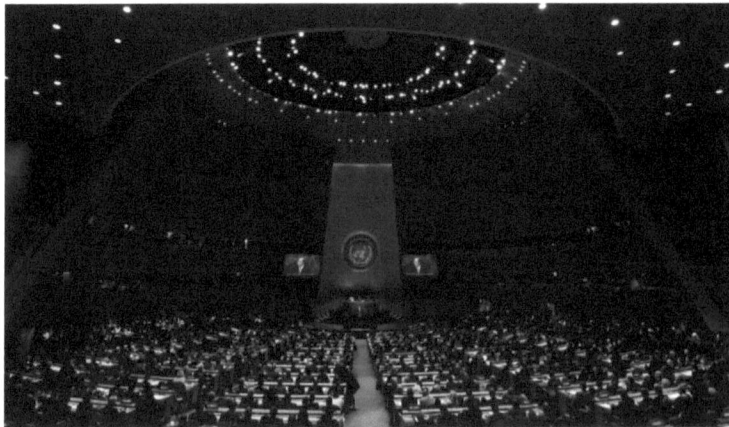

United Nations, AP Photo

The United Nations was created to prevent future wars and still exists today. Our healthy political, cultural, and economic relations with Japan are especially meaningful to me because I served in the Pacific during the war.

Photos by Mike & Lisa Becker

I am also happy to know that the people of Kwajalein still celebrate Liberation Day. Each year, on February 9th, there is a reenactment of the battle to free the Kwajalein people from Japanese occupation. They have a parade, races, ball games, and other festivities. These photos are from Liberation Day 2015 in Ebeye, Kwajalein. "We remember them today" was the 2015 theme for the celebration.

There are friendships and business partnerships that now bring us together in ways that would have been hard to believe back then. So many Americans live and work in Japan and many Japanese live and work in the United States. The same for Italy and Germany. It is incredibly inspiring.

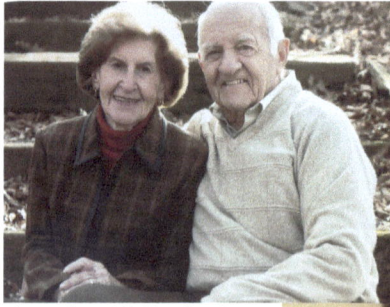
James E. and Bobbye Brooks

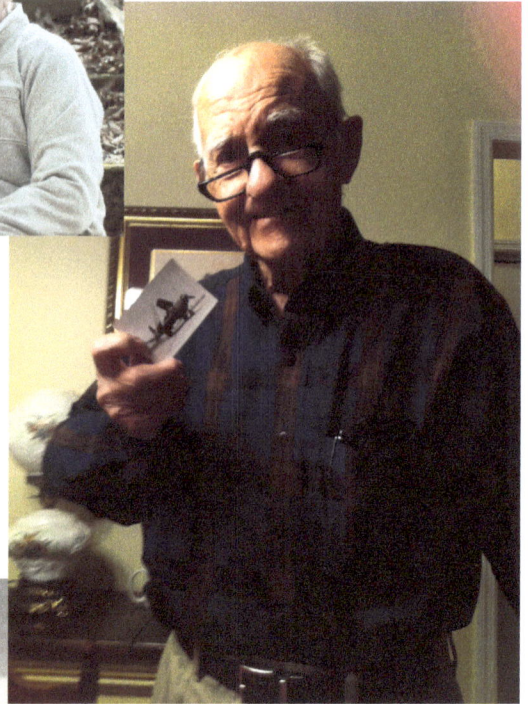
Photos, James E. Brooks

It is so difficult to speak of the enemy countries because we are such good friends today; it is a true testament of

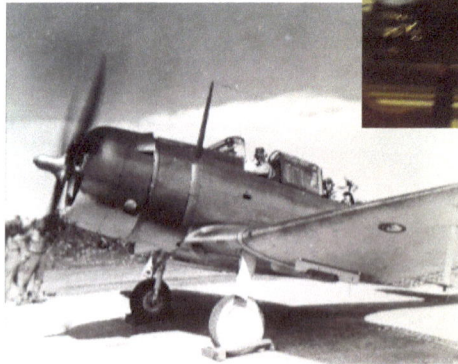
Taxiing planes on Kwajalein

the power of friendship. I've said before that it is important to remember what the war taught us. It's just amazing to think how far we've come in such a short time. I hope that good relations among all nations can continue for our children's sake.

Events leading up to WWII

World War One 1914–1918

The Great Depression 1929–1939

The Dust Bowl 1930s

Brief Timeline of WWII

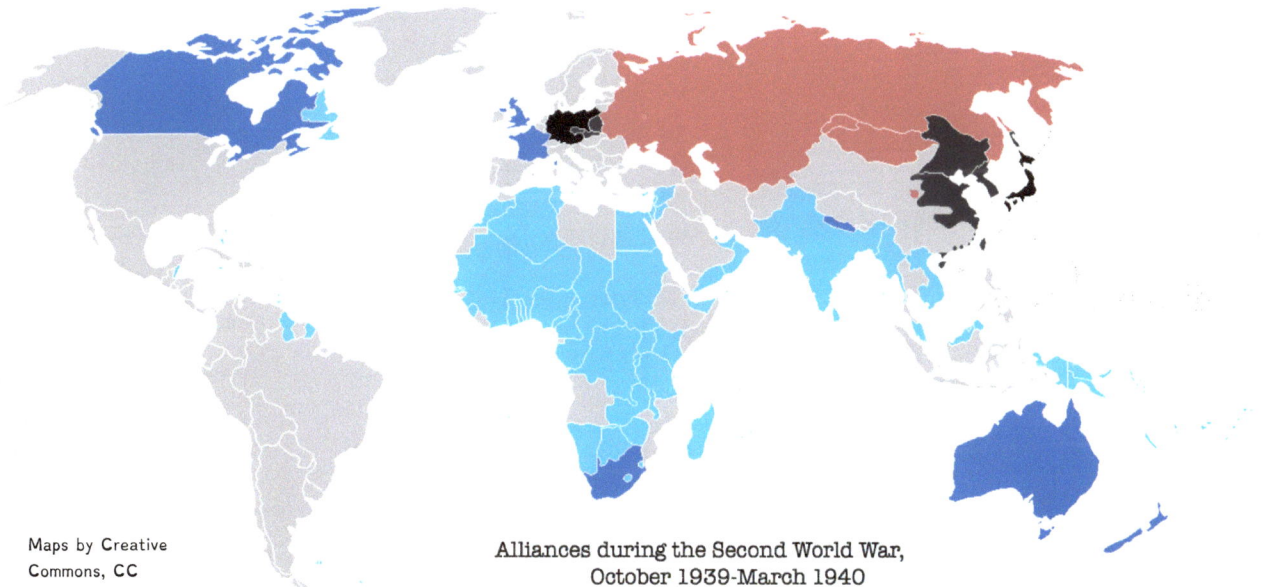

Maps by Creative
Commons, CC

Alliances during the Second World War,
October 1939-March 1940

- Western Allies (independent countries)
- Western Allies (colonies or occupied)
- Eastern Allies
- Axis (countries)
- Axis (colonies or occupied, including Vichy France)
- Neutral

October 2, 1935—May 1936 → Fascist Italy invades, conquers, and annexes Ethiopia.

October 25 → Nazi Germany and Fascist Italy sign a treaty of cooperation

November 1 1936 → the Rome-Berlin Axis is announced.

July 7, 1937 → Japan invades China, initiating World War II in the Pacific.

September 1, 1939 → Germany invades Poland, initiating World War II in Europe.

June 21 → Italy enters the war. Italy invades southern France.

October 1940 → Italy invades Greece from Albania on October 28.

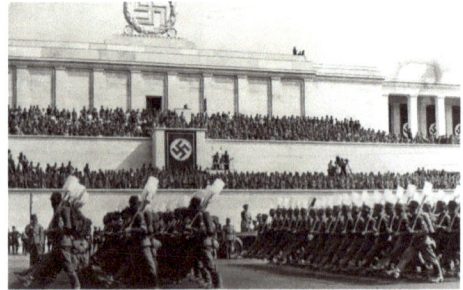

Adolf Hitler reviewing a Reich Labor Service (RAD) parade, Zeppelin Field, Nürnberg, Germany, Sep 1937

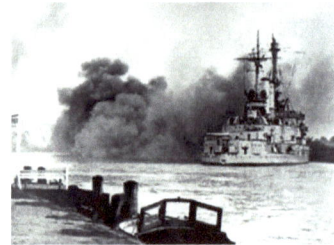

German Battleship attacks forts in Poland 1939

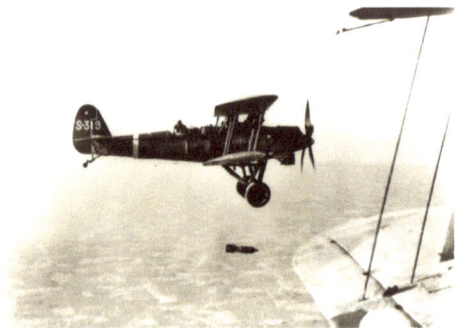

Japanese Army biplane dropping a bomb over China, 1937. Library of Congress

June 22, 1941–November 1941 →
Nazi Germany and its Axis partners
(except Bulgaria) invade the Soviet
Union.

December 7, 1941 → Japan bombs
Pearl Harbor.

December 8, 1941 → The United
States declares war on Japan,
entering World War II.

December 11–13, 1941 → Nazi
Germany and its Axis partners
declare war on the United States.

August–November 1942 → US troops
halt the Japanese island-hopping
advance towards Australia at
Guadalcanal in the Solomon Islands.
(1942 the year I was drafted into
WWII)

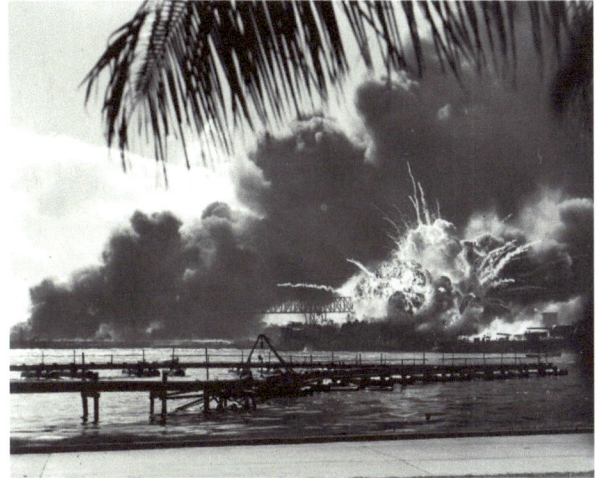

United States Destroyer USS Shaw being hit by
Japanese attack in Pearl Harbor Hawaii. December 7,
1941.

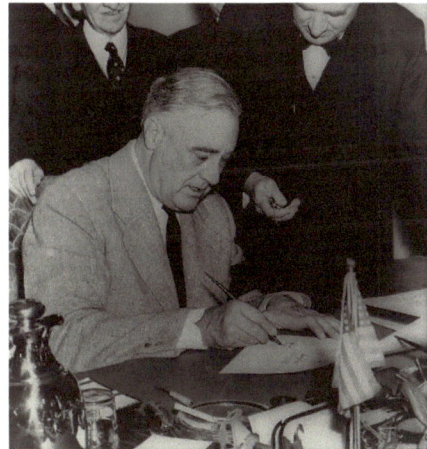

Franklin Roosevelt signing the Declaration of
War against Germany, 11 Dec 1941; Senator
Tom Connally stood by with watch to mark
exact time of declaration.
Library of Congress

June 6, 1944 → British and US troops successfully land on the Normandy beaches of France, opening a "Second Front" against the Germans.

August 20—25, 1944 → Allied troops reach Paris. On August 25, Free French forces, supported by Allied troops, enter the French capital. By September, the Allies reach the German border; by December, virtually all of France, most of Belgium, and part of the southern Netherlands are liberated.

December 16, 1944 → The Germans launch a final offensive in the west, known as the Battle of the Bulge, Allied forces along the German border. By January 1, 1945, the Germans are in retreat.

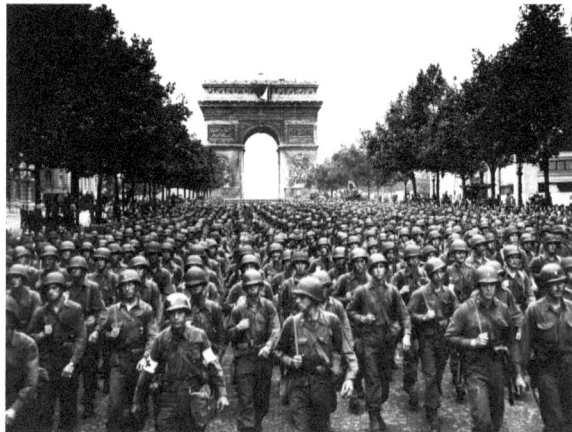

US Twenty-Eighth Infantry Division march along the Champs-Elysees, Paris, France with l'Arc de Triomphe in the background, Aug 29 1944. United States Army

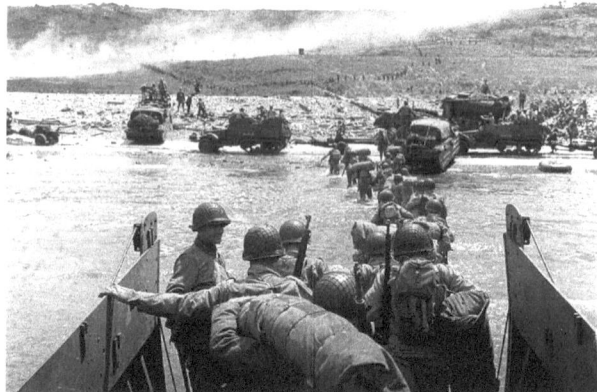

American troops waded ashore from a LCVP landing craft, Omaha Beach, Normandy, 6 Jun 1944. United States National Archives

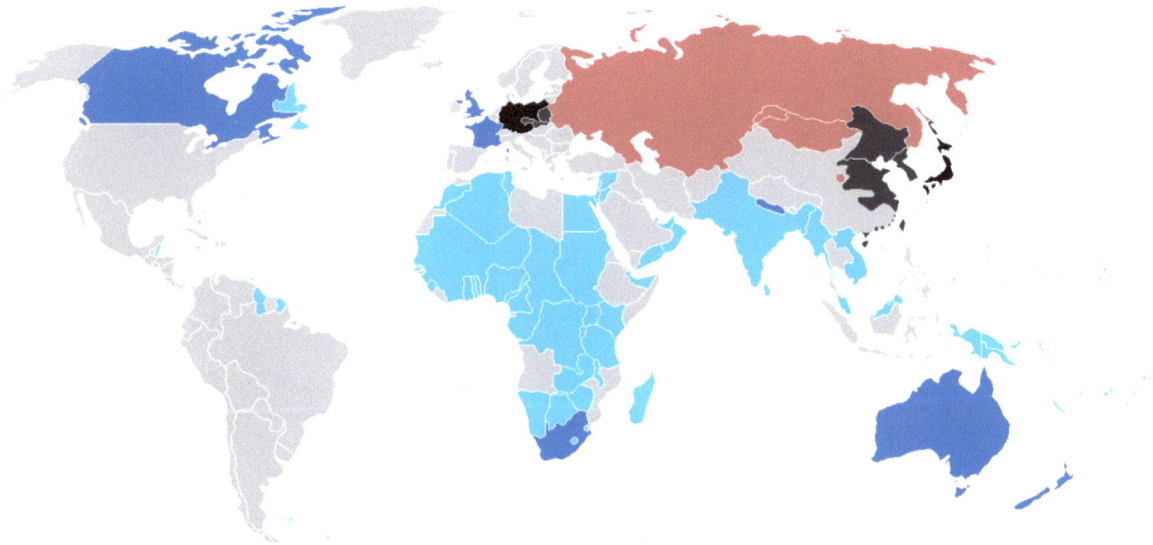

May 7, 1945 → Germany surrenders to the western Allies.

May 1945 → Allied troops conquer Okinawa, the last island stop before the Japanese Islands.

August 6, 1945 → The United States drops an atomic bomb on Hiroshima.

August 8, 1945 → The Soviet Union declares war on Japan and invades Manchuria.

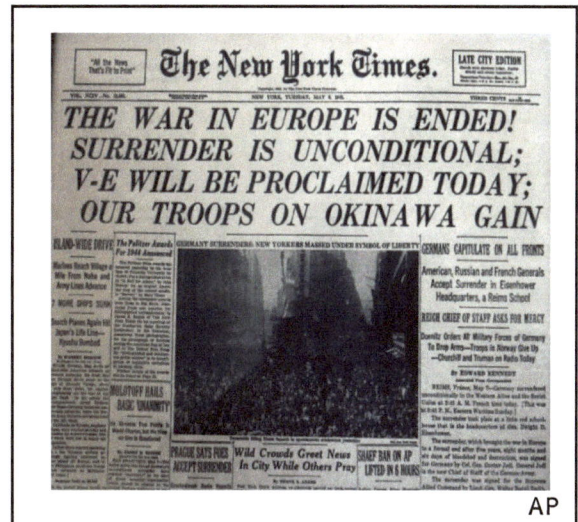

THE WAR IN EUROPE IS ENDED!
SURRENDER IS UNCONDITIONAL;
V-E WILL BE PROCLAIMED TODAY;
OUR TROOPS ON OKINAWA GAIN

AP

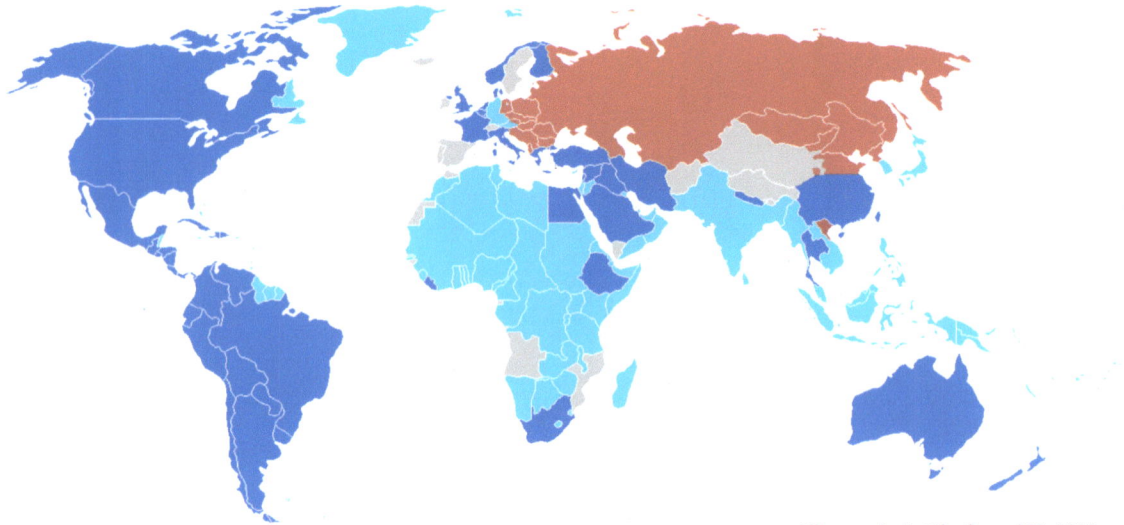

August 9, 1945 → The United States drops an atomic bomb on Nagasaki.

September 2, 1945 → Having agreed in principle to unconditional surrender on August 14, 1945, Japan formally surrenders, ending World War II.

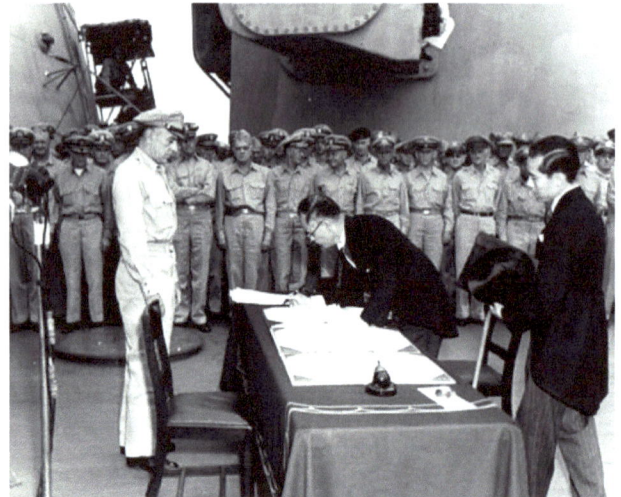

United States National Archives

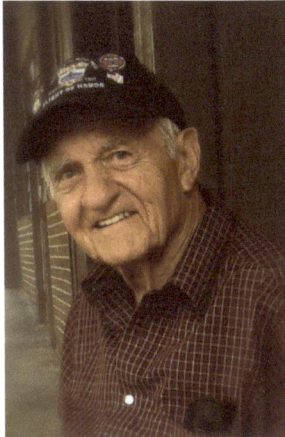

Remember to keep learning about WWII from books, memorials, movies, and museums. Being educated and aware helps you do your part in making our world better in small ways, and perhaps big ways too.
Take care of each other, Jimmy.

A note from Stephanie Fairchild Fister:

It is an honor and a privilege to listen to and write the words of James E. Brooks. I was born thirty-three years after the United States entered WWII and although I learned about the war in school and movies, it has been an altogether different lesson for me to hear about how the war affected the everyday lives of young people. His life is a good example of a young man living in a small town, going to school with friends, when global events interrupted his life and called him to do his part to save his country from invasion. It is an example in humanity's long struggle to make and keep power in the hands of the people, not a few leaders at the top. It is remarkable to listen to Jimmy at 89 years of age, and benefit from his vivid memories and wisdom.

James E. Brooks goes by the name Jimmy. He is well loved in his community. He did not keep in touch with his two friends with whom he shared a tent for over two years during the war. E.J. Otto and William "Willy" are listed in his book of notes he kept, but their addresses are difficult to read. Several of Jimmy's family members have worked to locate EJ and Willy but have been unable to find either of them or their families. It is likely that E.J. Otto was from Steelton, PA. Jimmy remembers that William's father was a set director for Warner Bros. in Hollywood, California. It may be that the last name of William's parents, Richard and Dorothy was Chadury or Charery. If you can help find these friends or their families please contact us.

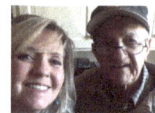

Stephanie Fairchild Fister
stephaniefairchildfister@gmail.com

Photographs taken by and owned by James E. Brooks are identified with his name.

Special thanks to Creative Commons for use of all maps marked CC, Creative Commons, Citing of their work is requested as follows:
    This work is licensed under the Creative Commons Attribution- ShareAlike 3.0 Unported License. To view a copy of this license, visit http://creativecommons.org/licenses/by-sa/3.0/ or send a letter to Creative Commons, PO Box 1866, Mountain View, CA 94042, USA.

Special thanks to National Archives and Records Administration for providing WWII photos.

Special thanks to the Associated Press for WWII photos.

Special thanks to the National for WWII photos.

Special thanks to Mike and Lisa Becker for permission and use the photographs of Kwajalein citizens celebrating Liberation Day 2015.

Special thanks to the Marine Bombing Squadron Six-Thirteen for permission and use of the photos from their website

Special thanks to these family members for additional proofing and editing!!
Nawanna Privett, Jennifer Brooks Griffith, Will Fister, Sha Fister, Hanna Fister, John Michael Griffith, Brian Griffith.

Additional copies of this book may be purchased on amazon.com

Information may be found on the website
whatsbestforourkids.com